Selected Topics in Blood Pressure Physiology

Edited by Aleksandar Kibel

Published in London, United Kingdom

Selected Topics in Blood Pressure Physiology
http://dx.doi.org/10.5772/intechopen.1002577
Edited by Aleksandar Kibel

Contributors
Abayomi Sanusi, Aleksandar Kibel, Amirali Ahrabi, Margarita Voitikova, Othman Beni Yonis, Raissa Khursa, Sepideh Poshtdar, Titus F. Msoka, Vedran Đambić

Notice
Statements and opinions expressed in the chapters are these of the individual contributors and not necessarily those of the editors or publisher. No responsibility is accepted for the accuracy of information contained in the published chapters. The publisher assumes no responsibility for any damage or injury to persons or property arising out of the use of any materials, instructions, methods or ideas contained in the book.

First published in London, United Kingdom, 2025 by IntechOpen
IntechOpen is the global imprint of INTECHOPEN LIMITED, registered in England and Wales, registration number: 11086078, 167-169 Great Portland Street, London, W1W 5PF, United Kingdom

For EU product safety concerns: IN TECH d.o.o., Prolaz Marije Krucifikse Kozulić 3, 51000 Rijeka, Croatia, info@intechopen.com or visit our website at intechopen.com.

British Library Cataloguing-in-Publication Data
A catalogue record for this book is available from the British Library

Selected Topics in Blood Pressure Physiology
Edited by Aleksandar Kibel
p. cm.

This title is part of the Physiology Book Series, Volume 30
Topic: Human Physiology
Series Editor: Tomasz Brzozowski
Topic Editor: Kunihiro Sakuma
Associate Topic Editor: Kotomi Sakai and Muneshige Shimizu

Print ISBN 978-1-83634-329-5
Online ISBN 978-1-83634-328-8
eBook (PDF) ISBN 978-1-83634-330-1
ISSN 2631-8261

If disposing of this product, please recycle the paper responsibly.

IntechOpen

intechopen.com

Built by scientists, for scientists

IntechOpen Book Series
Physiology
Volume 30

Aims and Scope of the Series

Modern physiology requires a comprehensive understanding of the integration of tissues and organs throughout the mammalian body, including the cooperation between structure and function at the cellular and molecular levels governed by gene and protein expression. While a daunting task, learning is facilitated by identifying common and effective signaling pathways mediated by a variety of factors employed by nature to preserve and sustain homeostatic life. As a leading example, the cellular interaction between intracellular concentration of $Ca+2$ increases, and changes in plasma membrane potential is integral for coordinating blood flow, governing the exocytosis of neurotransmitters, and modulating gene expression and cell effector secretory functions. Furthermore, in this manner, understanding the systemic interaction between the cardiovascular and nervous systems has become more important than ever as human populations' life prolongation, aging and mechanisms of cellular oxidative signaling are utilised for sustaining life. Altogether, physiological research enables our identification of distinct and precise points of transition from health to the development of multimorbidity throughout the inevitable aging disorders (e.g., diabetes, hypertension, chronic kidney disease, heart failure, peptic ulcer, inflammatory bowel disease, age-related macular degeneration, cancer). With consideration of all organ systems (e.g., brain, heart, lung, gut, skeletal and smooth muscle, liver, pancreas, kidney, eye) and the interactions thereof, this Physiology Series will address the goals of resolving (1) Aging physiology and chronic disease progression (2) Examination of key cellular pathways as they relate to calcium, oxidative stress, and electrical signaling, and (3) how changes in plasma membrane produced by lipid peroxidation products can affect aging physiology, covering new research in the area of cell, human, plant and animal physiology.

Meet the Series Editor

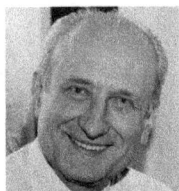

Prof. Dr. Thomas Brzozowski works as a professor of Human Physiology and is currently a Chairman at the Department of Physiology and is V-Dean of the Medical Faculty at Jagiellonian University Medical College, Cracow, Poland. His primary area of interest is physiology and pathophysiology of the gastrointestinal (GI) tract, with a major focus on the mechanism of GI mucosal defense, protection, and ulcer healing. He was a postdoctoral NIH fellow at the University of California and the Gastroenterology VA Medical Center, Irvine, Long Beach, CA, USA, and at the Gastroenterology Clinics Erlangen-Nuremberg and Munster in Germany. He has published 290 original articles in some of the most prestigious scientific journals and seven book chapters on the pathophysiology of the GI tract, gastroprotection, ulcer healing, drug therapy of peptic ulcers, hormonal regulation of the gut, and inflammatory bowel disease.

Meet the Volume Editor

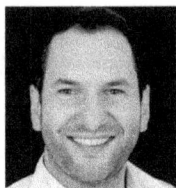

Aleksandar Kibel is an Associate Professor at the Department of Physiology and Immunology, Faculty of Medicine in Osijek and the Department of Clinical Medicine, Faculty of Dental Medicine and Health, University of Osijek, as well as a specialist in internal medicine and a subspecialist in cardiology at the International Medical Center Priora. He graduated from the Faculty of Medicine at the University of Osijek with an MD degree in 2009, achieving the maximum possible grade average. He completed his internship at the University Hospital Centre in Zagreb. He obtained his PhD in 2014 and later acquired the scientific grade of Senior Expert Associate in both Basic Medical Sciences and Clinical Medical Sciences. He has been engaged in preclinical and clinical scientific research for many years and has also participated in clinical trials. He was awarded the TOP scholarship for top students, the Faculty Council Award for exceptional academic success during medical school, and the Lions Club Award for the best students of the University, along with other awards for his activities at the Science Festival and the Osijek Medical Students' Day. He is the author of numerous scientific papers indexed in relevant databases (see CROSBI), author of book chapters and editor of a book on the renin-angiotensin system. He served as a guest editor and reviewer for the journals *Oxidative Medicine & Cellular Longevity* and *Journal of International Medical Research*, among others, and also reviewed and was a member of the editorial board for other foreign journals, including *Frontiers in Physiology*. He is a mentor for several graduate theses and is also a mentor for four doctoral students in the postgraduate doctoral program in Biomedicine and Health. He was the head of the institutional scientific research project IP-8 of the Faculty of Medicine, Osijek, and a collaborator on other scientific projects (including a project of the Croatian Science Foundation). He is the head of the MEFOS-2 research group of the Scientific Center of Excellence (ZCI) for personalized health care (in the Scientific Unit for Research, Production and Medical Testing of Functional Foods) and is also a member of the scientific board of the ZCI. He is the subject lead of Physiology and Pathophysiology at the University's Integrated Undergraduate and Graduate Study of Medicine in German, located at the Faculty of Medicine in Osijek. He is the Head of the Scientific Unit for Medical Research at the International Medical Center Priora.

Contents

Preface

Blood pressure regulation is a fundamental characteristic of the human circulatory system. As one of the most critical parameters of the cardiovascular system, arterial blood pressure must be precisely regulated, and this is achieved through a complex interplay of numerous regulatory mechanisms. Dysfunction of some of these regulatory networks may lead to inadequate blood pressure regulation, including states of elevated blood pressure and hypertension, which, over time, result in several serious consequences for the organism and damage to various tissues, contributing to morbidity and mortality.

The book *Selected Topics in Blood Pressure Physiology* aims to provide up-to-date insights into the regulation of arterial blood pressure and insights into regulatory dysfunction associated with hypertension.

The chapters will focus on hemodynamics and the fundamental mechanisms of blood pressure regulation, including the baroreceptor reflex, as well as mechanisms related to pressure natriuresis. Furthermore, chapters in the book will discuss a wide range of consequences that are connected to hypertension, which is a disorder that represents a significant public health burden, contributing to a decrease in life expectancy and a decrease in quality of life. The most important mechanisms of secondary hypertension will also be discussed. Finally, the book includes a chapter focusing on the effect of lifestyle changes on the regulation of arterial blood pressure.

We hope readers find the materials related to blood pressure physiology and hypertension interesting and that reading about these topics in this book facilitates further thought and research. We still have a long way to go to fully understand blood pressure physiology, especially at the functional, tissue, cellular, and molecular levels. This is essential for adequately treating elevated blood pressure and hypertension, as well as achieving future clinical goals, including reducing cardiovascular morbidity and mortality. This book is merely one of many "stepping stones" in this way and aims to contribute to disseminating knowledge and stimulating further research.

Aleksandar Kibel, M.D., Ph.D.
Associate Professor,
Internal Medicine Specialist,
Cardiology Subspecialist,
Head of the Scientific Unit for Medical Research,
International Medical Center Priora,
Čepin, Croatia

Faculty of Medicine,
Department of Physiology and Immunology,
J.J. Strossmayer University of Osijek,
Osijek, Croatia

Faculty of Dental Medicine and Health,
Department of Clinical Medicine,
J.J. Strossmayer University of Osijek,
Osijek, Croatia

Head of MEFOS2 Research Group of the Scientific Centre of Excellence
for Personalized Health Care,
J.J. Strossmayer University of Osijek,
Osijek, Croatia

Chapter 1

The Role of Baroreceptors in Blood Pressure

Amirali Ahrabi and Sepideh Poshtdar

Abstract

Baroreceptors are mechanoreceptors that play a crucial role in maintaining normal blood pressure and heart rate. There are two types of baroreceptors; arterial and cardiopulmonary. Arterial receptors are located in the carotid sinus and the aortic arch, while cardiopulmonary or volume baroreceptors are found within the atria, ventricles, and pulmonary vessels. Arterial baroreceptors are sensitive to vessel-wall stretching, and in cases of blood pressure alterations, impulses sent by these receptors reach the nucleus tractus solitarius, resulting in changes to heart rate, cardiac contractility, and peripheral vascular resistance. Cardiopulmonary baroreceptors provide information to the vagal center of the medulla regarding blood volume, thereby mediating changes in circulatory and renal function. In this chapter, we will delve into the physiology, mechanisms of function, clinical significance, and emerging research related to baroreceptors.

Keywords: baroreceptor, baroreflex, blood pressure, carotid sinus, hypertension, nucleus tractus solitarius

1. Introduction

Various sensors within the body continuously monitor arterial pressure. Whenever arterial pressure deviates from its normal range, several reflex responses are activated, including the baroreceptor reflex (baroreflex). This reflex helps adjust cardiac output and total peripheral resistance to restore arterial pressure to its normal level.

In the short term, within seconds to minutes, these adjustments are achieved through the pivotal activity of autonomic nerves affecting the heart and peripheral vessels. Over the long term, spanning hours to days, other mechanisms, such as blood volume regulation involving renal processes assist these baroreceptors in maintaining arterial pressure.

A disruption of the baroreflex can lead to significant blood pressure (BP) dys-regulation, resulting in increased BP variability. This may include sudden drops in pressure when moving from a lying to a standing position, along with abnormal spikes in pressure, which heighten the risk of life-threatening events such as heart attacks and strokes. This chapter provides an in-depth exploration of the physiologic anatomy of baroreceptors, their role in blood pressure regulation, and the importance of baroreflex sensitivity. We further examine how the central nervous system interprets baroreflex signals, the clinical significance of baroreflex function, and how its impairment contributes to various diseases.

2. Physiologic anatomy

Baroreflex helps the circulatory system adjust to changing conditions in daily life, keeping BP, heart rate, and blood volume within a stable physiological range. The baroreceptors are nerve endings that are stimulated by stretching. There are two main types: arterial and cardiopulmonary baroreceptors (which will be discussed later in this chapter).

Arterial baroreceptors are mechanoreceptors that can sense arterial pressure from the stretches of elastic arterial walls. This mechanosensing is mediated through the activation of PIEZO1 and PIEZO2 ion channels [1]. These baroreceptors are densely located in two areas: (1) the carotid sinus, which is slightly cephalad the bifurcation of the carotid artery, and (2) the wall of the aortic arch. Notably, these baroreceptors rarely can be found in other cervical and thoracic arteries.

Carotid baroreceptors send their impulses through a small branch of nerves, named Hering's nerve or carotid sinus nerve, to the glossopharyngeal nerves in the neck. On the other hand, baroreceptors of the aortic arch transmit their signals to the vagus nerves through a branch of nerves called the aortic depressor nerve. The final destination of all these signals is the nucleus tractus solitarius (NTS) located in the medullary area of the brain stem (**Figure 1**). The NTS integrates input from multiple other sources, including chemoreceptors (both peripheral and central), renal mechanoreceptors and chemoreceptors (*via* renal afferent nerves), muscle ergoreceptors, respiratory neurons, and neurons from the cortex and hypothalamus.

The neural interconnections between this region, other parts of the medullary circulation center, and higher centers such as the hypothalamus and the cortex are intricate and not yet fully understood. Nonetheless, it is established that the glossopharyngeal and vagus nerves excite the NTS by releasing glutamate. In response, the NTS excites the caudal ventrolateral medulla's (CVLM) neurons by releasing glutamate. CVLM in turn releases the inhibitory neurotransmitter γ-aminobutyric acid (GABA) to the rostral ventrolateral medulla (RVLM), subsequently decreasing the activity of preganglionic sympathetic neurons. Additionally, excitatory projections from the NTS reach cardiac preganglionic parasympathetic neurons, so-called vagal motor neurons, located in the nucleus ambiguus and the dorsal motor nucleus.

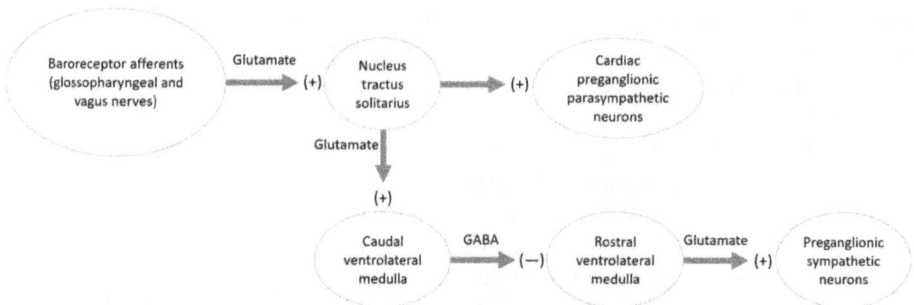

Figure 1.
The baroreceptor pathway connecting baroreceptor afferent signals to sympathetic and parasympathetic responses.

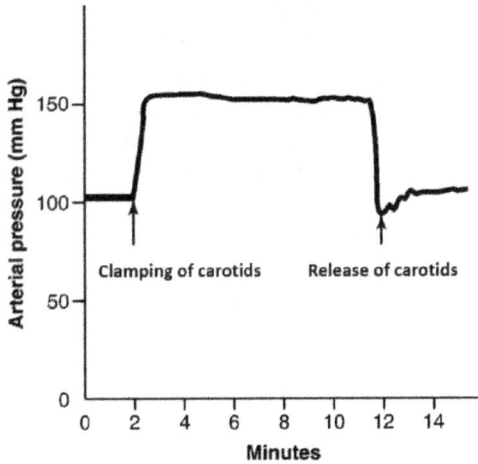

Figure 2.
Effect of bilateral carotid artery clamping on baroreflex activity and subsequent change in arterial pressure.

The arterial baroreflex has a widespread impact on the entire body. When stimulated by elevated arterial pressure, the baroreflex increases, leading to a decrease in sympathetic activity and an increase in parasympathetic activity. The overall effects are as follows: (1) vasodilation of veins and arterioles throughout the peripheral circulatory system, leading to a decrease in end-diastolic volume, and (2) a reduction in both heart rate and the strength of heart contractions, resulting in an increase in end-systolic volume. The latter also protects the heart from lethal arrhythmias. Consequently, the baroreflex decreases the arterial pressure through reduced peripheral resistance and lower cardiac output.

In contrast, low arterial pressure produces the opposite effects, reflexively prompting an increase in pressure back toward normal levels. Another example is physical exercise, where an increase in BP is necessary to ensure adequate blood perfusion to the muscles. This rise is facilitated by the attenuation of baroreflex activity, as maintaining maximal reflex function would prevent the required pressure elevation. To achieve this, the activation of skeletal muscle afferent fibers through contraction or stretching raises the baroreceptor threshold pressure, thereby restricting its reflex activity [2].

Figure 2 shows the effect of carotid sinus baroreceptors on arterial pressure after bilaterally clamping the carotid arteries. During the occlusion, arterial pressure remains elevated; however, it drops sharply upon the removal of the clamps. The initial overcompensation is then gradually readjusted to normal levels within a minute after the clamps are released.

3. Changes in arterial pressure and its effect on baroreceptors

Arterial baroreceptors are stimulated not only by the absolute stretch of the arterial wall but also by variations in this stretch, that is, changes in arterial pressure. Animal studies have shown that two types of baroreceptors exist in the carotid sinus, each with distinct properties [3, 4]. Type I baroreceptors, primarily A-fiber myelinated axons, play a key role in stabilizing arterial pressure, while type II baroreceptors, consisting of C-fiber unmyelinated and small A-fiber myelinated axons, are implicated in signaling the absolute level of arterial pressure. Type I baroreceptors undergo resetting for this purpose, which refers to a shift in their response to stimuli, whereas type II baroreceptors have higher threshold pressures and do not reset, as discussed below. Therefore, both mean arterial pressure and pulse pressure are key determinants of arterial baroreceptor activity. It is important to note that functional differences in the central processing of these two types of baroreceptors have not yet been determined.

As shown in **Figure 3**, the carotid baroreceptors are inert in arterial pressures below 50 mm Hg but begin to elicit activity around 50 mmHg and reach a maximum plateau in approximately 180–200 mm Hg of arterial pressure. In lower pressures, this activity is only during the systolic phase of the cardiac cycle but extends to the remaining diastolic part around 100 mm Hg of arterial pressure. The aortic arch baroreceptors act similarly at arterial pressure levels that are about 30 mm Hg higher.

A decrease in systemic arterial pressure leads to a reduction in baroreflex, resulting in a compensatory increase in BP and cardiac output. Conversely, an increase in pressure causes the arterioles to dilate, which reduces cardiac output until BP returns to its original baseline level.

It is noteworthy that the most sensitivity of these baroreceptors is in the range of normal BP, that is, 100 mmHg. Even small changes to the arterial pressure in this region cause the baroreceptor feedback mechanism to regulate and readjust pressure back to normal levels. Another important point is that baroreceptors are far more responsive to rapid fluctuations in BP than to prolonged sustained high levels of BP.

The baroreceptor system is referred to as a pressure buffer system because it counteracts variations in arterial pressure. The nerves associated with the baroreceptors are also known as buffer nerves. A study conducted by Cowley et al. [5] demonstrated that the 24-hour variation in arterial BP is significantly greater in baroreceptor-denervated dogs compared to normal dogs. They concluded that the main role of the baroreflex is not to establish the chronic level of arterial BP but rather to reduce fluctuations in systemic arterial BP. These fluctuations can arise from excitement, daily rhythms, eating, defecation, noises, or other unknown origins.

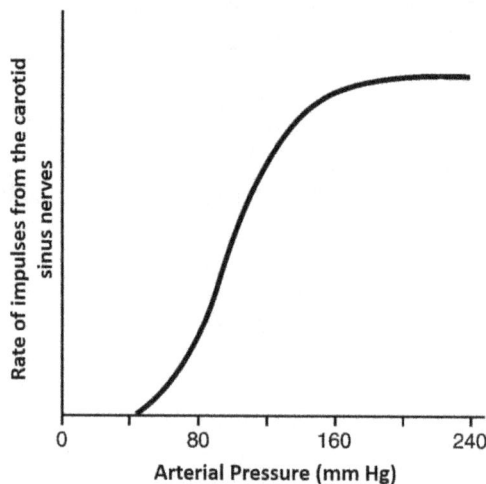

Figure 3.
Baroreflex activity, measured by impulses sent through the carotid sinus nerves, in different arterial pressures.

Another example of arterial pressure adjustments by baroreceptors is the sudden change in body posture when standing up after lying down. The sudden drop in arterial pressure in the head could lead to loss of consciousness as soon as a person stands up. However, the drop in pressure detected by the baroreceptors triggers an immediate reflex, causing a strong sympathetic response throughout the body that helps to reduce this decline in pressure. The impairment of the baroreflex leads to a significant drop in BP, which will be discussed in more detail later.

4. Baroreflex sensitivity

To quantify the effect of baroreflex, baroreflex sensitivity (BRS) is introduced by scientists. BRS is mathematically defined as the change in the inter-beat interval in milliseconds per unit change in BP. For example, if the interval between heartbeats increases by 100 milliseconds while BP rises by 10 mmHg, the BRS is calculated as 100/10, resulting in a value of 10 milliseconds per mmHg. Decreased BRS increases BP variability, which in turn further diminishes BRS, creating a vicious cycle. Two points are worth noting: first, this index reflects the baroreflex's effect on the sinus node rather than its BP buffering capacity; second, it does not specify whether the changes in the inter-beat interval in response to BP fluctuations are mainly caused by increased or decreased sympathetic or parasympathetic activity [6].

BRS measurement is regarded as a valuable tool for assessing various cardiovascular diseases [7]. It specifically evaluates the autonomic system's ability to respond to BP changes at the aortic arch and carotid sinus [8]. BRS function is also affected by several risk factors, with obesity being a major one. Obesity significantly lowers BRS, leading to sympathovagal imbalance by decreasing parasympathetic activity and increasing SNA [9]. High abdominal visceral fat, in particular, has been linked to reduced BRS. Additionally, conditions related to obesity, such as diabetes [10], and hypertension [11], as well as independent factors like aging [12], sex [13], and physical activity [14], can also disrupt the balance between the sympathetic and parasympathetic nervous systems.

5. Various interpretations of baroreflex signals by the CNS

The baroreflex is one of the main apparatuses of CNS that can help to ascertain the proper blood flow to the different organs. Interestingly, central parts of the baroreflex pathway, especially NTS, CVLM, and RVLM, can modulate the activity of this reflex to an organ-specific response, primarily through region-specific changes in sympathetic nerve activity (SNA). Although the precise mechanisms by which these nuclei interact to produce region-specific changes in SNA, or whether they dynamically adjust their networks, are not yet fully understood, it is clear that these effects are mediated by shifts in the baroreflex action curve, which is processed within these nuclei to generate targeted changes in SNA [15]. The purpose of these adjustments is the optimal regulation of arterial pressure.

For instance, during freezing behavior, an innate response of animals to threats or potential dangers like predators, studies show that renal sympathetic nerve activity (RSNA) increases by up to 1.5 times, while lumbar sympathetic nerve activity (LSNA) remains still [16]. Heart rate decreases, allowing the animal to conserve energy for a potential transition from freezing to the fight-or-flight phase. With the decrease in heart rate and the subsequent decline in cardiac output (Cardiac Output = Stroke Volume × Heart Rate), the increased RSNA helps maintain arterial pressure by raising peripheral resistance (recall that Mean Arterial Pressure = Cardiac Output × Total Peripheral Resistance). The purpose of retaining intact LSNA, which primarily innervates the muscles of the lower extremities, is to preserve blood flow to these muscles in case of a fight-or-flight response, as LSNA is negatively correlated with muscle blood flow. These region-specific adjustments in the baroreflex curves appear to reflect a highly advanced survival strategy.

Another example of CNS control over the baroreflex curve occurs during sleep phases. During the non-rapid eye movement (NREM) phase, both RSNA and LSNA, as well as heart rate and arterial pressure, decrease. Of particular interest is that during rapid eye movement (REM) sleep—a phase where brain activity rises to wakeful levels—RSNA paradoxically decreases, while LSNA significantly increases [17]. As previously mentioned, this is a direct effect of the brain's upper control centers on the baroreflex curve, prioritizing blood flow to the CNS, kidneys, and splanchnic organs due to their higher metabolic demands during this phase, while reducing muscle blood flow through increased LSNA [15]. In summary, baroreflex pathways may be distinctly separated, enabling selective modifications of baroreflex action curves that result in differential changes in sympathetic nerve activity.

6. Long-term regulation of arterial pressure

There have been controversies regarding the long-term effect of baroreceptors on arterial pressure. Some studies in the twentieth century indicated that these receptors can adapt to elevated arterial pressure levels within 1–2 days, suggesting that they may not play a significant role in the long-term regulation of BP [18–20]. For instance, when BP abruptly rises, baroreceptors initially send a high frequency of signals. However, this rate decreases significantly within a few minutes. Over the following 1–2 days, the rate continues to decline, ultimately returning to near-normal levels despite the persistently elevated BP. Conversely, when BP drops drastically, baroreceptors initially cease sending signals but gradually resume firing, approaching their normal rate over a period of 1–2 days. This demonstrates the baroreceptor's adaptation to long-term changes in BP. However, two points should be noted about these studies. First, due to experimental limitations, previous studies extrapolated short-term recordings of baroreceptor afferent nerves to assess the long-term effects of these receptors in chronic states, where the acute setting may not accurately represent the body's long-term BP regulation. Second, these studies did not account for the potential plasticity of the vasomotor center in their conclusions. While the adaptation to prolonged high arterial pressure may be partially attributed to the resetting of arterial mechanoreceptors, changes in central circulatory regulation also play a pivotal role [21, 22]. As described by Schreihofer et al. [23] in the chronic absence of baroreceptor input, the RVLM still controls activity SNA to regulate arterial pressure. Furthermore, even without continuous excitatory input from the NTS, glutamatergic signals in baroreceptor-denervated rats activate the CVLM, which persistently inhibits the RVLM.

Contrary to previous assumptions, experimental studies suggest that baroreceptors maintain some degree of sensitivity even after prolonged BP changes [24]. This ongoing sensitivity may contribute to long-term BP regulation, particularly by influencing the activity of the sympathetic nerve in the kidneys. Barrett et al., in their study assessing the effect of baroreceptors on RSNA, concluded that in sinoaortic-denervated rabbits, where baroreceptor afferent signals were severed, RSNA did not change with angiotensin II infusion. However, a significant decrease in RSNA was observed in sham-operated rabbits [25]. Accordingly, the activity of the renal sympathetic nerve depends on the baroreflex. When arterial pressure remains elevated for an extended period, baroreflexes can reduce RSNA, leading to greater sodium and water excretion. Additionally, renin secretion is also inhibited as a result of the suppression of RSNA [19]. These processes gradually reduce blood volume, aiding arterial pressure to return to normal levels.

In summary, the baroreflex alone is not sufficient for the long-term regulation of arterial pressure, and therefore, baroreceptors must work in conjunction with other systems to effectively regulate mean arterial pressure over the long term.

7. Cardiopulmonary baroreceptors

Cardiopulmonary baroreceptors, also known as low-pressure receptors, are found in the atria and pulmonary arteries. Their function is yet to be completely understood, but they are similar to that of arterial baroreceptors and help to reduce BP variations by responding to changes in blood volume. Although the cardiopulmonary baroreceptors are unable to sense systemic arterial pressure directly, they are sensitive to concurrent increases in pressure within low-pressure regions of the circulation due to increased blood volume. These receptors initiate reflexes that complement the arterial baroreflex, thereby enhancing the overall reflex system's efficacy in regulating arterial pressure.

When the atria are stretched due to the increase in blood volume or central venous pressure, the activation of low-pressure atrial baroreceptors triggers a reflex that reduces sympathetic nerve signals to the kidneys, decreases fluid reabsorption in the renal tubules, and dilates the afferent arterioles in the kidneys. The dilation of the afferent arterioles additionally leads to an increase in glomerular capillary pressure, which in turn raises the amount of fluid filtered into the kidney tubules. Simultaneously, signals from these baroreceptors are sent to the hypothalamus to reduce the secretion of antidiuretic hormone (ADH) and subsequent reduction in water reabsorption in tubules. Another hormone released upon activation of atrial baroreceptors is atrial natriuretic peptide (ANP), which promotes the excretion of sodium and water, thereby helping to reduce blood volume levels back to normal. The ultimate outcome of this mechanism—improved glomerular filtration and reduced fluid reabsorption—is a decrease in the elevated blood volume. Decreased blood volume or central venous pressure initiates the exact opposite mechanism.

8. Bainbridge reflex

An increase in atrial pressure can raise the heart rate, particularly when the heart rate is initially slow. The atrial mechanoreceptors that activate the Bainbridge reflex send afferent signals *via* the *vagus* nerves to the medulla in the brain. From there, efferent signals are sent back through the *vagal* and sympathetic nerves, increasing both heart rate and the strength of heart contractions. This reflex helps prevent the accumulation of blood in the circulatory system, particularly in the veins, atria, and pulmonary circulation.

When the heart rate is already fast, atrial stretching from fluid infusion may reduce the heart rate by triggering arterial baroreceptors. As a result, the overall effect of increased blood volume and atrial stretch on heart rate depends on the interplay between arterial baroreflexes, which tend to decrease heart rate, and the Bainbridge reflex, which works to increase it. When blood volume is above normal levels, the Bainbridge reflex frequently raises the heart rate, even though the arterial baroreflexes act against it.

9. Diseases with baroreflex impairment

Neurons of the baroreflex can be damaged by neurodegenerative, metabolic, autoimmune, traumatic, or toxic mechanisms. Any lesion in the baroreflex pathway, including afferent, central, or efferent neurons, can cause BP fluctuations and lead to hypo- or hyperperfusion in different organs. Diseases involving baroreflex failure can be divided into three main categories:

9.1 Efferent baroreflex failure

Baroreflex efferent neurons are predominantly damaged by diabetes, followed by synucleinopathies, such as pure autonomic failure, Parkinson's disease, dementia with Lewy bodies, and multiple-system atrophy. Clinically, this disorder is characterized by a sustained drop in BP of at least 20/10 mm Hg within 3 minutes of standing upright. In some patients, however, the BP drop is delayed and occurs after prolonged standing. The primary pathophysiology involves the inhibition of norepinephrine release at the neurovascular junction, leading to inadequate vasoconstriction during standing or physical exertion. This results in the observed orthostatic hypotension and symptoms of organ hypoperfusion, such as dizziness, lightheadedness, blurred vision, and syncope.

Over half of these patients experience supine hypertension (BP >140/90 mm Hg), likely due to the activation of residual sympathetic fibers and denervation supersensitivity, a condition that is associated with target organ damage in chronic cases [26]. Additionally, extracellular fluid volume regulation is also disrupted, especially at night, leading to increased renal excretion of sodium and water, which worsens orthostatic hypotension in the morning.

Efferent baroreflex dysfunction can be an early indicator of synucleinopathies, allowing for diagnosis before typical motor or cognitive symptoms appear. Studies show that patients with isolated efferent baroreflex failure have a 10% annual risk of developing Parkinson's disease, Lewy body dementia, or multiple system atrophy [27]. Treatment includes educating the patient, addressing aggravating factors (e.g., dehydration, medications), using postural maneuvers, and employing pharmacologic measures to increase intravascular volume and peripheral resistance.

9.2 Afferent baroreflex failure

The acquired form of afferent baroreflex failure is observed in patients with a history of radiotherapy or radical surgery in the cervical region, as well as in patients with rare tumors affecting the NTS. Iatrogenic causes may also include procedures like carotid endarterectomy or angioplasty, leading to damage either to the baroreceptors themselves or to the afferent fibers, vagal, or glossopharyngeal nerves. Familial dysautonomia (the Riley–Day syndrome) is the congenital form of afferent baroreflex failure.

In the absence of afferent nerve signaling to the NTS, this nucleus cannot inhibit the premotor sympathetic neurons in the RVLM. As a result, unleashed sympathetic activation leads to norepinephrine release, causing vasoconstriction, tachycardia, elevated BP and its variability, headaches, flushing, and agitation. In some cases, orthostatic hypotension is also detected. Given that afferent baroreflex is compromised in the Guillain–Barré syndrome, these patients experience severe fluctuations in BP but nearly invariant heart rate.

9.3 Cardiovascular autonomic disorders without detectable nerve disease

The most common impairments in the baroreflex pathway occur without any detectable nerve pathology. Conditions such as vasovagal syncope and postural tachycardia syndrome fall into this category.

9.3.1 Vasovagal syncope

Syncope is a temporary loss of consciousness and postural tone caused by a brief general cerebral hypoperfusion, which resolves spontaneously without any lasting neurological effects. Vasovagal syncope, reaching a prevalence of 16% among the population [28], is stimulated by a reflex that causes activation of parasympathetic and inhibition of sympathetic. It can be stimulated by central factors, such as emotions, pain, or blood phobia, or by peripheral factors, like prolonged standing or increased activity of carotid sinus afferents. The use of diuretics or vasodilators, including alcohol, marijuana, and alpha-blockers, can increase susceptibility. The baroreflex plays a crucial role in controlling cardiac vagal tone and, if activated inappropriately, can significantly inhibit heart function, resulting in a severe decrease in heart rate or even asystole. Sudden and inappropriate activation of the baroreflex can cause syncope due to the drastic decrease in sympathetic activity and intense cardioinhibition by increased parasympathetic activity. However, the specific afferent nerve pathways and central nervous system mechanisms responsible for reflex syncope are still poorly understood.

9.3.2 Postural tachycardia syndrome

This syndrome is diagnosed by a sustained increase in heart rate of at least 30 beats per minute (or 40 beats per minute in the pediatric population) within 10 minutes of standing, accompanied by symptoms of sympathetic activation such as palpitations, shortness of breath, chest pain, and anxiety. In this syndrome, BP does not decrease upon standing. The severity of symptoms does not correlate with heart rate, and reducing tachycardia often does not relieve the symptoms. Various mechanisms have been proposed for postural tachycardia syndrome, including baroreflex impairment, hyperventilation, cardiac atrophy, intravascular volume dysregulation, and defects in the cardiac norepinephrine transporter [29–31].

10. Clinical significance of baroreflex

The role of the baroreflex in regulating arterial pressure has prompted research into chronic electrical stimulation devices designed to precisely control afferent signals to the central nervous system in patients with resistant hypertension or those with heart failure. Animal studies have shown promising results, as electrical stimulation of the carotid sinus in dogs led to a reduction in whole-body norepinephrine spillover, α1-adrenergic receptor activity, mean arterial BP, and heart rate without increase in plasma renin activity [24]. First carotid sinus electrical stimulation in humans was performed in 1967 [32]. In the past few years, the prototype Rheos system (CVRx, Minneapolis, MN) was introduced, in which the baroreflex is stimulated by implanting electrodes in the perivascular space surrounding each carotid sinus, with the leads connected to a pulse generator. This device can be fully programmed using a radio-frequency-based external system, allowing adjustments to parameters such as intensity, frequency, and pulse duration throughout the day. However, its requirement for bilateral surgery may pose a drawback for broader adoption in clinical practice. A more recent version of this device, the Barostim Neo (CVRx, Minneapolis, MN), is attached to the surface of the carotid sinus with sutures and is implanted unilaterally. Numerous studies have been completed or are ongoing to assess the safety and efficacy of these devices, comparing their outcomes to standard medical management in patients with resistant hypertension and those with symptomatic heart failure (EF > 40%) [33–37]. For instance, an observational study found that implantation of the Barostim Neo system in patients with drug-resistant hypertension significantly reduced office BP (systolic: −25 ± 33 mmHg, diastolic: −9 ± 18 mmHg; n = 50) and 24-hour ambulatory BP (systolic: −8 ± 23 mmHg, diastolic: −5 ± 13 mmHg; n = 46) at 24 months. The median number of antihypertensive medications per patient also decreased from seven to five [38]. In the double-blind, sham-controlled US Rheos Pivotal trial, 265 patients with drug-resistant hypertension (office BP ≥160/80 mmHg and 24-hour ambulatory systolic BP ≥135 mmHg) had the Rheos device implanted and were randomly assigned (2:1) to either immediate baroreflex activation therapy or delayed therapy after 6 months (control group). After 6 months, office BP reduction was significantly greater in the immediate treatment group compared to the control group (−26 ± 30 mmHg vs. −17 ± 29 mmHg, P = 0.03). Interestingly, a subsequent study concluded that unilateral, particularly right-sided, stimulation of carotid baroreceptors has a more significant impact on reducing BP compared to bilateral or left-sided stimulation [39]. The reductions in BP following acute baroreflex activation were accompanied by decreased heart rate, muscle sympathetic nerve activity, and plasma renin concentration, suggesting that the response was mediated by sympathetic inhibition and enhanced parasympathetic activity [40]. These effects also counteract the sympathetic overactivation and parasympathetic withdrawal commonly seen in heart failure patients. The HOPE4HF and BeAT-HF trials demonstrated that baroreflex activation therapy using the Barostim Neo system, when combined with medical treatment, significantly improved outcomes in patients with heart failure with reduced ejection fraction (LVEF ≤35%) and NYHA functional class III, compared to medical therapy alone [41, 42]. Improvements were seen in walk distance, quality of life, NYHA functional class, and natriuretic peptide levels. Additionally, there was a trend toward fewer hospital stays due to heart failure. With over 94% of patients experiencing no major neurological, cardiovascular, or procedure-related complications, the safety of baroreflex activation therapy was also confirmed. So far, these results represent an exciting potential addition to the clinician's armament in the fight against chronic arterial hypertension and heart failure.

Another innovative device is the MobiusHD stent (Vascular Dynamics), which induces a pulsatile increase in vessel wall stretch and amplifies the baroreflex, thereby sustainably suppressing SNA. It is implanted endovascularly on one side in the proximal internal carotid artery [43]. In the first-in-human, noncontrolled, open-label CALM-FIM_EUR study, 30 patients received the MobiusHD stent at six European centers [44].

After 6 months, significant reductions were observed in both office and 24-hour ambulatory BP. Additionally, the median number of antihypertensive medications and daily doses had decreased. Although the results were promising, serious adverse events, including hypotension, worsening hypertension, and intermittent claudication, were unfortunately reported in the study. Further randomized, sham-controlled trials are needed to evaluate the efficacy of this treatment and to carefully weigh its benefits against potential complications associated with its minimally invasive implantation.

11. Conclusion

In this chapter, we discussed the physiology of the baroreflex and its role in both blood pressure buffering and cardioprotection. Previous reports primarily focused on this buffering in response to acute changes in blood pressure, but we also highlighted the evolving paradigm of the baroreflex's role in chronic blood pressure regulation. Two recent concepts have also been covered: (1) baroreflex sensitivity (BRS) and its implications in cardiovascular diseases, which can be altered by various medical conditions, and (2) different aspects of the CNS response to the baroreflex curve, along with the subsequent region-specific changes in sympathetic nerve activity. Finally, we reviewed diseases associated with baroreflex impairment and the growing body of evidence on the clinical significance of interventions targeting baroreflex activity to treat conditions such as resistant hypertension and heart failure.

Conflict of interest

The authors declare no conflict of interest.

Author details

Amirali Ahrabi[1,2*] and Sepideh Poshtdar[2,3]

1 Sina Trauma and Surgery Research Center, Tehran University of Medical Sciences, Tehran, Iran

2 School of Medicine, Tehran University of Medical Sciences, Tehran, Iran

3 Eye Research Center, Farabi Eye Hospital, Tehran University of Medical Sciences, Tehran, Iran

*Address all correspondence to: aa.ahrabi@gmail.com

IntechOpen

References

[1] Zeng WZ, Marshall KL, Min S, Daou I, Chapleau MW, Abboud FM, et al. PIEZOs mediate neuronal sensing of blood pressure and the baroreceptor reflex. Science. 2018;**362**(6413):464-467. DOI: 10.1126/science.aau6324

[2] Di Rienzo M, Parati G, Radaelli A, Castiglioni P. Baroreflex contribution to blood pressure and heart rate oscillations: Time scales, time-variant characteristics and nonlinearities. Philosophical Transactions of the Royal Society A. 1892;**2009**(367):1301-1318. DOI: 10.1098/rsta.2008.0274

[3] Seagard JL, Gallenberg LA, Hopp FA, Dean C. Acute resetting in two functionally different types of carotid baroreceptors. Circulation Research. 1992;**70**(3):559-565. DOI: 10.1161/01. res.70.3.559

[4] Seagard JL, Hopp FA, Drummond HA, Van Wynsberghe DM. Selective contribution of two types of carotid sinus baroreceptors to the control of blood pressure. Circulation Research. 1993;**72**(5):1011-1022. DOI: 10.1161/01. RES.72.5.1011

[5] Cowley AW, Liard JF, Guyton AC. Role of the baroreceptor reflex in daily control of arterial blood pressure and other variables in dogs. Circulation Research. 1973;**32**(5):564-576. DOI: 10.1161/01. RES.32.5.564

[6] Swenne CA. Baroreflex sensitivity: Mechanisms and measurement. Netherlands Heart Journal. 2013;**21**(2):58-60. DOI: 10.1007/ s12471-012-0346-y

[7] Al-Khateeb AA, Limberg JK, Barnes JN, Joyner MJ, Charkoudian N, Curry TB. Acute cyclooxygenase

inhibition and baroreflex sensitivity in lean and obese adults. Clinical Autonomic Research. 2017;**27**(1):17-23. DOI: 10.1007/s10286-016-0389-z

[8] Pankova NB, Alchinova IB, Cherepov AB, Yakovenko EN, Karganov MY. Cardiovascular system parameters in participants of arctic expeditions. International Journal of Occupational Medicine and Environmental Health. 2020;**33**(6):819-828. DOI: 10.13075/ijomeh.1896.01628

[9] Konstantinidou SK, Argyrakopoulou G, Tentolouris N, Karalis V, Kokkinos A. Interplay between baroreflex sensitivity, obesity and related cardiometabolic risk factors (review). Experimental and Therapeutic Medicine. 2022;**23**(1):67. DOI: 10.3892/ etm.2021.10990

[10] Kück JL, Bönhof GJ, Strom A, Zaharia OP, Müssig K, Szendroedi J, et al. Impairment in baroreflex sensitivity in recent-onset type 2 diabetes without progression over 5 years. Diabetes. 2020;**69**(5):1011-1019. DOI: 10.2337/ db19-0990

[11] Guyenet PG, Stornetta RL, Souza G, Abbott SBG, Brooks VL. Neuronal networks in hypertension: Recent advances. Hypertension. 2020;**76**(2):300-311. DOI: 10.1161/ hypertensionaha.120.14521

[12] Serhiyenko VA, Serhiyenko AA. Cardiac autonomic neuropathy: Risk factors, diagnosis and treatment. World Journal of Diabetes. 2018;**9**(1):1-24. DOI: 10.4239/wjd.v9.i1.1

[13] Fu Q, Ogoh S. Sex differences in baroreflex function in health and disease. The Journal of Physiological Sciences.

2019;**69**(6):851-859. DOI: 10.1007/
s12576-019-00727-z

[14] Fukuma N, Kato K, Munakata K, Hayashi H, Kato Y, Aisu N, et al. Baroreflex mechanisms and response to exercise in patients with heart disease. Clinical Physiology and Functional Imaging. 2012;**32**(4):305-309. DOI: 10.1111/j.1475-097X.2012.01127.x

[15] Miki K, Ikegame S, Yoshimoto M. Regional differences in sympathetic nerve activity are generated by multiple arterial baroreflex loops arranged in parallel. Frontiers in Physiology. 2022;**13**:858654. DOI: 10.3389/fphys.2022.858654

[16] Kondo N, Yoshimoto M, Ikegame S, Miki K. Differential shifts in baroreflex control of renal and lumbar sympathetic nerve activity induced by freezing behaviour in rats. Experimental Physiology. 2021;**106**(10):2060-2069. DOI: 10.1113/ep089742

[17] Yoshimoto M, Yoshida I, Miki K. Functional role of diverse changes in sympathetic nerve activity in regulating arterial pressure during REM sleep. Sleep. 2011;**34**(8):1093-1101. DOI: 10.5665/sleep.1168

[18] Cowley AW Jr. Long-term control of arterial blood pressure. Physiological Reviews. 1992;**72**(1):231-300. DOI: 10.1152/physrev.1992.72.1.231

[19] Lohmeier TE, Iliescu R. The baroreflex as a long-term controller of arterial pressure. Physiology (Bethesda, Md.). 2015;**30**(2):148-158. DOI: 10.1152/physiol.00035.2014

[20] Malpas SC. Sympathetic nervous system overactivity and its role in the development of cardiovascular disease. Physiological Reviews. 2010;**90**(2):513-557. DOI: 10.1152/physrev.00007.2009

[21] Cavalleri MT, Burgi K, Cruz JC, Jordão MT, Ceroni A, Michelini LC. Afferent signaling drives oxytocinergic preautonomic neurons and mediates training-induced plasticity. American Journal of Physiology. Regulatory, Integrative and Comparative Physiology. 2011;**301**(4):R958-R966. DOI: 10.1152/ajpregu.00104.2011

[22] Sved AF, Schreihofer AM, Kost CK Jr. Blood pressure regulation in baroreceptor-denervated rats. Clinical and Experimental Pharmacology & Physiology. 1997;**24**(1):77-82. DOI: 10.1111/j.1440-1681.1997.tb01787.x

[23] Schreihofer AM, Ito S, Sved AF. Brain stem control of arterial pressure in chronic arterial baroreceptor-denervated rats. American Journal of Physiology. Regulatory, Integrative and Comparative Physiology. 2005;**289**(6):R1746-R1755. DOI: 10.1152/ajpregu.00307.2005

[24] Lohmeier TE, Iliescu R, Dwyer TM, Irwin ED, Cates AW, Rossing MA. Sustained suppression of sympathetic activity and arterial pressure during chronic activation of the carotid baroreflex. American Journal of Physiology. Heart and Circulatory Physiology. 2010;**299**(2):H402-H409. DOI: 10.1152/ajpheart.00372.2010

[25] Barrett CJ, Guild SJ, Ramchandra R, Malpas SC. Baroreceptor denervation prevents sympathoinhibition during angiotensin II-induced hypertension. Hypertension. 2005;**46**(1):168-172. DOI: 10.1161/01.HYP.0000168047.09637.d4

[26] Fanciulli A, Jordan J, Biaggioni I, Calandra-Buonaura G, Cheshire WP, Cortelli P, et al. Consensus statement on the definition of neurogenic supine hypertension in cardiovascular autonomic failure by the American autonomic society (AAS) and the

European Federation of Autonomic Societies (EFAS): Endorsed by the European academy of neurology (EAN) and the European Society of Hypertension (ESH). Clinical Autonomic Research. 2018;**28**(4):355-362. DOI: 10.1007/s10286-018-0529-8

[27] Kaufmann H, Norcliffe-Kaufmann L, Palma JA, Biaggioni I, Low PA, Singer W, et al. Natural history of pure autonomic failure: A United States prospective cohort. Annals of Neurology. 2017;**81**(2):287-297. DOI: 10.1002/ana.24877

[28] Salari N, Karimi Z, Hemmati M, Mohammadi A, Shohaimi S, Mohammadi M. Global prevalence of vasovagal syncope: A systematic review and meta-analysis. Global Epidemiology. 2024;**7**:100136. DOI: 10.1016/j.gloepi.2024.100136

[29] Stewart JM, Pianosi P, Shaban MA, Terilli C, Svistunova M, Visintainer P, et al. Postural hyperventilation as a cause of postural tachycardia syndrome: increased systemic vascular resistance and decreased cardiac output when upright in all postural tachycardia syndrome variants. Journal of the American Heart Association. 2018;**7**(13):e008854. DOI: 10.1161/JAHA.118.008854

[30] Shibata S, Fu Q, Bivens TB, Hastings JL, Wang W, Levine BD. Short-term exercise training improves the cardiovascular response to exercise in the postural orthostatic tachycardia syndrome. The Journal of Physiology. 2012;**590**(15):3495-3505. DOI: 10.1113/jphysiol.2012.233858

[31] Shannon JR, Flattem NL, Jordan J, Jacob G, Black BK, Biaggioni I, et al. Orthostatic intolerance and tachycardia associated with norepinephrine-transporter deficiency. The New England Journal of Medicine. 2000;**342**(8):541-549. DOI: 10.1056/nejm200002243420803

[32] Rothfeld EL, Parsonnet V, Raman KV, Zucker IR, Tiu R. The effect of carotid sinus nerve stimulation on cardiovascular dynamics in man. Angiology. 1969;**20**(4):213-218. DOI: 10.1177/000331976902000405

[33] Scheffers IJ, Kroon AA, Schmidli J, Jordan J, Tordoir JJ, Mohaupt MG, et al. Novel baroreflex activation therapy in resistant hypertension: Results of a European multi-center feasibility study. Journal of the American College of Cardiology. 2010;**56**(15):1254-1258. DOI: 10.1016/j.jacc.2010.03.089

[34] Economic Evaluation of Baroreceptor STIMulation for the Treatment of Resistant HyperTensioN (ESTIM-rHTN). 1 Sept 2022. Available from: https://clinicaltrials.gov/study/NCT02364310 [Accessed: September 20, 2024]

[35] BAROSTIM NEO Hypertension Pivotal Trial. 1 July 2024. Available from: https://clinicaltrials.gov/ct2/show/NCT01679132 [Accessed: September 20, 2024]

[36] Heusser K, Tank J, Brinkmann J, Menne J, Kaufeld J, Linnenweber-Held S, et al. Acute response to unilateral unipolar electrical carotid sinus stimulation in patients with resistant arterial hypertension. Hypertension. 2016;**67**(3):585-591. DOI: 10.1161/hypertensionaha.115.06486

[37] Lohmeier TE, Iliescu R. Chronic lowering of blood pressure by carotid baroreflex activation: Mechanisms and potential for hypertension therapy. Hypertension. 2011;**57**(5):880-886. DOI: 10.1161/hypertensionaha.108.119859

[38] Wallbach M, Born E, Kämpfer D, Lüders S, Müller GA, Wachter R, et al. Long-term effects of baroreflex activation therapy: 2-year follow-up data of the BAT neo system. Clinical Research in Cardiology. 2020;**109**(4):513-522. DOI: 10.1007/s00392-019-01536-5

[39] de Leeuw PW, Alnima T, Lovett E, Sica D, Bisognano J, Haller H, et al. Bilateral or unilateral stimulation for baroreflex activation therapy. Hypertension. 2015;**65**(1):187-192. DOI: 10.1161/hypertensionaha.114.04492

[40] Heusser K, Tank J, Engeli S, Diedrich A, Menne J, Eckert S, et al. Carotid baroreceptor stimulation, sympathetic activity, baroreflex function, and blood pressure in hypertensive patients. Hypertension. 2010;**55**(3):619-626. DOI: 10.1161/hypertensionaha.109.140665

[41] Zile MR, Lindenfeld J, Weaver FA, Zannad F, Galle E, Rogers T, et al. Baroreflex activation therapy in patients with heart failure with reduced ejection fraction. Journal of the American College of Cardiology. 2020;**76**(1):1-13. DOI: 10.1016/j.jacc.2020.05.015

[42] Abraham WT, Zile MR, Weaver FA, Butter C, Ducharme A, Halbach M, et al. Baroreflex activation therapy for the treatment of heart failure with a reduced ejection fraction. Netherlands Heart Journal. 2015;**3**(6):487-496. DOI: 10.1016/j.jchf.2015.02.006

[43] van Kleef M, Bates MC, Spiering W. Endovascular Baroreflex amplification for resistant hypertension. Current Hypertension Reports. 2018;**20**(5):46. DOI: 10.1007/s11906-018-0840-8

[44] Spiering W, Williams B, Van der Heyden J, van Kleef M, Lo R, Versmissen J, et al. Endovascular baroreflex amplification for resistant hypertension: A safety and proof-of-principle clinical study. Lancet. 2017;**390**(10113):2655-2661. DOI: 10.1016/s0140-6736(17)32337-1

Chapter 2

Pressure Natriuresis in Blood Pressure Control

Vedran Đambić and Aleksandar Kibel

Abstract

The kidneys play an important role in controlling arterial blood pressure by regulating extracellular fluid volume, through excretion of sodium and water, which is called pressure natriuresis, or diuresis. Sodium and water homeostasis is controlled by the integrated physiological functions of organ systems, including renal mechanisms, but also with an influence of the renal and non-renal sympathetic nervous system and the endocrine system (renin-angiotensin-aldosterone system, cardiac natriuretic peptides, antidiuretic hormone, and oxytocin). Pressure natriuresis represents the basal level for arterial blood pressure dysregulation. The imbalance of complex renal and non-renal hemodynamic and neurohumoral mechanisms leads to the disruption of antidiuretic mechanisms, which results in the development of arterial hypertension. Knowledge of all mechanisms enables an integrated understanding of the regulation of arterial blood pressure, which is a key step in the targeted and individual treatment of one of the most common diseases today.

Keywords: pressure natriuresis, diuresis, arterial blood pressure, kidneys, sodium, renin-angiotensin-aldosterone system, sympathetic nervous system, cardiac natriuretic peptides, hypertension

1. Introduction

The kidneys manage blood pressure by regulating the volume of extracellular fluid through the primary excretion of sodium and the secondary excretion of water through osmosis [1].

After a systemic increase in blood pressure, there is an increase in renal perfusion pressure, which results in the inhibition of renal tubular reabsorptive mechanisms and increased excretion of sodium and water to return blood pressure to normal, which is called pressure natriuresis, that is, diuresis [1, 2].

Pressure natriuresis is the main, non-adaptive mechanism with infinite gain responsible for long-term control of blood pressure with the goal of daily full compensation of blood pressure fluctuations [1].

2. Insight into the mechanism of pressure natriuresis

Sodium homeostasis is controlled by the integrated physiological functions of organ systems including the hemodynamic (peripheral and renal arteries) and neurohumoral systems (renal sympathetic nerves, renal autacoids, renin-angiotensin-aldosterone system, cardiac natriuretic peptides, antidiuretic hormone, and oxytocin) [3, 4].

The blood pressure value in the body is the point at which pressure natriuresis and the volume of extracellular fluid are in balance [2]. An increase in blood pressure leads to an increase in renal perfusion pressure (RPP). An increase in shear stress in the preglomerular vasculature due to autoregulatory vasoconstriction in response to rise in RPP activates endothelial nitric oxide synthase and NO production, increased release of prostaglandin E2 and renal kinins, and a decrease in intrarenal angiotensin II in the outer medulla, resulting in an increase in medullary blood flow (MBF) as a result of reduced vascular resistance of renal medulla arteries mediated by guanosine $3',5'$-cyclic monophosphate (cGMP) and protein kinase G [1, 2]. An increase in medullary blood flow (MBF) due to renal encapsulation leads to an increase in renal interstitial hydrostatic pressure (RIHP, 40% contribution to the mechanism of pressure natriuresis) around the vasa recta, which disturbs the balance of Starling forces. Thus, changes in pressure natriuresis do not significantly affect glomerular filtration rate (GFR) because the afferent myogenic response and the tubuloglomerular feedback mechanism effectively keep GFR constant over a wide range of systolic blood pressure levels [2].

The key driver of pressure natriuresis is increased RIHP leading to antagonism of paracellular passive osmotic reabsorption of sodium and water in the proximal tubule and loop of Henle and causing rapid redistribution of sodium/hydrogen transporter isoform 3 (NHE3) out of the apical brush border along with inhibition of basolateral Na^+K^+-ATPase (NKA) in the proximal tubule [2, 5]. NHE3 in the proximal tubule reabsorbs ~65% of filtered Na^+ [2]. It is expressed in all segments of the nephron, except for the macula-dense and intercalated cells of the distal nephron [6]. The sodium/chloride cotransporter (NCC) in the apical membrane of the distal convoluted tubule (DCT) participates in salt reabsorption [7]. The epithelial Na + channel (ENaC) plays a key role in the absorption of Na^+ in the collecting duct of the kidney, the expression of which is significantly increased by aldosterone and vasopressin [8]. Sodium-dependent Pi cotransporters (2 Na-Pi), especially the type 2 Na-Pi cotransporter, include three cotransporter isoforms that are expressed on the brush membrane of the renal proximal tubules and enhance the excretion of not only phosphate but also sodium, as demonstrated by immunoblotting of NHE3 knockout mice [9]. In the basolateral membrane of renal epithelial cells, there is Na^+K^+-ATPase, which is not only well known as an ion pump but also a new class of receptors associated with the Src family kinase signaling pathway. Increased renal perfusion pressure resulting in increased endogenous cGMP activates the Src pathway, resulting in internalization and inactivation of NKA and decreased expression and activity of (NHE-3), thereby reducing Na^+ reabsorption [10]. $Na^+K^+2Cl^-$ cotransporter class 2 (NKCC2) is localized on the apical membrane of the epithelial cells of the thick ascending limb of the loop of Henle and the macula densa and is responsible for ~20–25% of NaCl reabsorption and modulates the preglomerular resistance of the afferent arteriole and the secretion of renin from granule cells of the juxtaglomerular apparatus (JGA) [11]. Na^+ glucose transporters (SGLT1 and SGLT2) are located in the proximal tubule of the nephron, which also contributes to sodium reabsorption (SGLT2 transports Na^+ and glucose in a 2:1 ratio, while SGLT2 transports in a 1:1 ratio) [6].

As mentioned, during the increase in renal perfusion pressure, there is also the release of paracrine factors (renal autocoids) that lead to the activation or inhibition of pro-natriuretic and antinatriuretic mediators. The main paracrine modulators of pressure natriuresis are angiotensin II (Ang II), 20-hydroxyeicosatetraenoic acid (20-HETE, metabolite of arachidonic acid produced by cytochrome P450), nitric oxide (NO), prostaglandin E2, renal kinins, adenosine triphosphate (ATP), endothelin 1, medullary O_2^- and H_2O_2. Paracrine factors significantly contribute to the redistribution of the NHE3 transporter, the internalization of the distal tubule sodium/chloride cotransporter, and the internalization of the type 2 Na-Pi cotransporter into cytoplasmic vesicles in microvilli [4].

The main antinatriuretic mediators are Ang II, aldosterone, HETE and Antidiuretic hormone (ADH) [4]. The main indirect effect of Ang II is a decrease in peritubular capillary pressure and an increase in Na transport. The direct action is realized through the angiotensin receptor (AT1 receptor) in the kidney, increasing the activity of NHE3 (but not Na-Pi cotransporter type 2) in the microvilli, the Na^+Cl^- cotransporter in the distal tubule and ENaC in the collecting duct [12, 13]. Angiotensin III (Ang III) mediated activation of angiotensin II receptor type 2 (AT 2 R) *via* protein phosphatase 2A (PP2A), bradykinin, nitric oxide, and cGMP signaling cascade results in increased natriuresis [14]. Aldosterone acts on mineralocorticoid receptors located in the distal tubule and collecting duct of the nephron, increasing Na reabsorption and potassium excretion through Na/ENaCs and potassium channels by NKA [4]. HETEs prevent NHE3 redistribution, Na-Pi cotransporter type 2 internalization, and inhibition of the basolateral NKA. Medullary O_2^- and H_2O_2 reduce the natriuretic response to increased RPP by a currently unknown mechanism [2]. ADH is extremely sensitive to the increase in Na concentration in the plasma and achieves its antinatriuretic (antidiuretic) effect *via* the V2 receptor in the kidney by increasing the reabsorption of water in the collecting duct of the nephron through the formation of aqueous aquaporin 2 (AQP2) and by increasing the number of ENaCs in the thick ascending limb that reabsorbs Na^+ [4]. The V1a receptor mediates the pro-natriuretic effect by inhibiting the renal reabsorption of Na in the connecting tubules and collecting ducts [4]. Oxytocin achieves its natriuretic effects directly by increasing the rate of glomerular filtration and decreasing tubular reabsorption of Na, and indirectly by cardiac excretion of Atrial natriuretic peptide (ANP), as well as by reducing the polydipsia response by acting on the tuberomammillary nucleus [4, 15].

The pro-natriuretic effect of NO manifests through the inhibition of sodium reabsorption in the PCT and the thick ascending limb of Henle and in the collecting duct by acting on the $Na^+K^+2Cl^-$ cotransporter and the Na^+/H exchanger. Prostaglandin E2 inhibits sodium reabsorption in the PCT and in the collecting duct and, as a potent vasodilator in the medulla, suppresses the vasoconstrictor effects of intrarenal Ang II [4]. Endothelin-1 has natriuretic effects mediated through the dilation of renal blood vessels *via* the endothelin receptor (ETA) receptor, while endogenous stimulation of ETB in the kidney exerts antinatriuretic effects *via* renal tubular NO, cGMP, and protein kinase G signaling [16]. ANP and B-type natriuretic peptide (BNP) act on the natriuretic peptide receptor A (NPR-A) inducing vasodilation of the afferent glomerular arteriole and vasoconstriction of the efferent glomerular arteriole (increasing the glomerular filtration rate) and reducing the activity of the cation channel that mediates electrogenic Na absorption to exert its pro-natriuretic effect [4]. Purinergic signaling also contributes to the regulation of natriuresis *via* a metabotropic GPCR (P2Y 2 receptor) whose activation *via* ATP and uridine-5'-triphosphate (UTP) increases sodium excretion by blocking ENaC [17]. Also, intracellular calcium and free oxygen radicals can significantly increase the expression of ENaC in oxidative stress [18]. The renal dopaminergic system inhibits sodium transport in all segments of the nephron and causes at least 50% of renal sodium excretion in conditions of moderate sodium excess [19]. Dopamine receptor-1 (D1R) activation inhibits luminal transport of sodium ions (NHE3, NaPi-Iic), while activation inhibits NKA activity and increases NHE3 degradation *via* USP-mediated ubiquitinylation [19].

Inhibitors of the sodium-glucose cotransporter 2 (SGLT2) of increased glucose excretion increase diuresis and natriuresis by reducing sodium reabsorption in the most proximal segments of the renal tubule and additionally inhibit the sodium-hydrogen exchanger 3, but due to strong counter-regulatory responses that are associated with the regulation of vasopressin, aldosterone, ketoglutarate, uromodulin, and carbonic anhydrase, any natriuretic or osmotic diuretic effect of SGLT2 inhibitors was canceled [6, 20, 21].

3. Influence of sympathetic nervous system activity on pressure natriuresis

The activity of the sympathetic nervous system contributes significantly to the long-term control of arterial blood pressure. Excessive activity of renal sympathetic nerves changes renal hemodynamics, urinary sodium excretion, and renin secretion. Afferent (sensory) information originates from arterial baroreceptors (in the carotid sinus and aortic arch) and peripheral organs (including the kidneys). Afferent fibers of the renal sympathetic nervous system are located within the wall of the renal pelvis in the interlobular and arcuate arteries and, to a lesser extent, around the interlobular arteries and afferent arterioles [1]. Afferent fibers travel to the nucleus tractus solitarius (NTS) and paraventricular nucleus of the hypothalamus, where they integrate and result in activation of the caudal ventrolateral medulla (CVLM) and rostral ventrolateral medulla (RVLM). RVLM efferent neurons project to sympathetic preganglionic neurons in the spinal cord [22]. Neural projections exit the spinal cord (intermediolateral column of the spinal cord, from T6 to L2 segments) *via* ventral horns and synapses of sympathetic preganglionic fibers (paravertebral chain or aorticorenal, celiac, superior mesenteric ganglia). Postganglionic nerves enter the renal hilus along the renal arteries and veins and branch around the vasculature of the cortex and medulla of the kidney (α1A-adrenoreceptor) to the granular cells of the juxtaglomerular apparatus (β1-adrenoreceptors) and the basal membrane of the tubular epithelial cells inside the nephron (α 1A - and α 1B -adrenoreceptors). The main neurotransmitters of afferent fibers are substance P and a peptide related to the calcitonin gene, while that of efferent fibers is noradrenaline [1]. Renal sympathetic nerves directly regulate natriuresis by regulating renal β1-adrenergic receptors, resulting in renin release, and stimulating renal α1-adrenergic receptors, resulting in sodium reabsorption [23]. By vasoconstricting the afferent and efferent arterioles, the sympathetic nervous system directly proportionally reduces renal blood flow (RBF) and glomerular filtration. It causes an increase in renin secretion by activating the JGA, which leads to the activation of the RAAS. In the proximal tubules, catecholamines activate the basolateral NKA and increase NHE3 activity, allowing the entry of Na^+ from the tubule lumen into the epithelial cells (increasing sodium and water reabsorption). Low-intensity stimulation of the sympathetic nervous system leads to only renin secretion, while the decrease in RBF and GFR was observed only at the highest levels of renal sympathetic nerve activity, which leads to a significant decrease in pressure natriuresis [1].

In addition to the baroreflex mediated by sympathetic nervous activity, there are additional mechanisms mediated by baroreceptor activation in the control of pressure natriuresis. Increased levels of circulating ANP contribute to increased sodium excretion and decreased blood pressure. Activation of baroreceptors leads to a decrease in cardiac output and an increase in cardiac pressure, which stretches the walls of the atria, resulting in the release of ANP. ANP provides a central link between the heart and kidney that mediates increased natriuresis during chronic baroreflex activation. ANP represents a compensatory mechanism for increasing natriuresis in the absence of renal sympathoinhibition, which speaks in favor of the cooperative redundancy of these two mechanisms [1].

The reno-renal reflex is formed by the activation of mechanosensory afferent nerves, which leads to reflex inhibition of the ipsi- and contralateral activity of the efferent sympathetic nerve of the kidney and consequent increased compensatory natriuresis with a significant contribution to the regulatory network of sodium and water homeostasis. An increase in the activity of the efferent renal sympathetic nerve enhances the activity of the afferent renal sympathetic nerve, while the increased afferent activity inhibits the efferent activity by negative feedback of the reno-renal reflex (prevents excessive activation of the renal sympathetic nerves and sodium retention). This mechanism is activated after sodium or fluid overload. However, there are pathological conditions (e.g., some forms of chronic kidney disease, renal artery stenosis, or phenol-induced kidney damage) in which this inhibitory reflex is impaired, resulting in a vicious cycle of increased sympathetic activity with a consequent increase in arterial blood pressure. It is important to emphasize that at the level of the nucleus tractus solitarius (NTS) and the paraventricular nucleus of the hypothalamus, input information triggered by baroreceptors is integrated with renal afferent signals, to obtain an integrated reference response of the renal sympathetic nerve. In the absence of an afferent innervation signal, baroreceptors cannot influence efferent sympathetic renal activity [1].

Mechanical deformation of nerve endings (increased pressure in the pelvis, i.e., during urine flow), changes in the chemical composition of urine, renal ischemia and renal pain are the main stimuli of afferent renal sympathetic nerve fibers [24].

Arterial hypertension must be understood as a complex balance of renal (and non-renal) mechanisms, among which is increased sympathetic nervous activity, which can be a primary change or a secondary one. Therefore, knowledge of the mechanisms of renal sympathetic nerve activity modulation is of key importance for the treatment of especially resistant hypertension [1].

4. Factors contributing to changes in pressure natriuresis

Chronically changing pressure natriuresis is a complex regulatory system at the kidney level that controls the basal level of blood pressure and contributes to the regulation of blood pressure within the normotensive or hypertensive range. Chronic hypertension can occur in case of a disorder of this long-term mechanism, which has the capacity for potentially boundless gain and non-adaptive performance. In hypertensive individuals, pressure natriuresis is less effective than in normotensive individuals across the entire blood pressure range, and therefore a higher blood pressure is required to achieve sodium balance. Hypertension can therefore only occur as a result of a primary shift in the intrinsic mechanisms linking blood pressure to natriuresis or disruption of modulators of this relationship. The relationship between specific blood pressure levels and corresponding natriuresis (and diuresis) is defined by the PN curve, the position and shape of which are determined by all the components that participate in sodium reabsorption, whose function is impaired in different pathophysiological scenarios. Mechanisms that promote sodium reabsorption (i.e., decrease sodium excretion) shift the PN curve to the right (leading to arterial hypertension, since a higher BP is necessary for each level of natriuresis), while mechanisms that decrease sodium reabsorption (i.e., increase sodium excretion) shift the curve to the left [1].

In hypertension, the mechanism of pressure natriuresis is abnormal because sodium excretion is the same as in normotension despite elevated arterial pressure [2]. Combined effects of transient increase in blood pressure, oxidative stress, inflammation, local vasoconstriction, chronic kidney disease, nephron loss, bilateral renal artery stenosis, salt retention, high salt intake, increased renal sympathetic activity, lack of nitric oxide in the kidneys, adverse effects of drugs on the kidneys and inefficient use of diuretics can lead to disturbances of pressure natriuresis and shift the pressure curve to the right [1, 2].

Cytokines can modulate salt and water balance by causing endothelial dysfunction, altering sympathetic tone, and/or increasing sodium transport along the nephron [25]. The main responsible cytokines affecting natriuresis are synthesized by pro-inflammatory T helper 1 and T helper 17 cells and M1 macrophages, namely tumor necrosis factor (TNF), interleukin 17A, interleukin 1 and interferon (IFN) [25].

Interestingly, therapeutic enlargement of renal lymphatic vessels (lymphangiogenesis) in mice increases natriuresis and lowers blood pressure under conditions of sodium retention [26].

5. Changes in pressure diuresis in salt-sensitive subjects

Salt sensitivity refers to a physiological characteristic in humans (and in animal models) in which blood pressure changes in parallel with changes in salt intake. Sodium homeostasis and salt sensitivity are not only associated with renal dysfunction but also with endothelial dysfunction, which may perhaps be connected to the accumulation of osmotically inactive sodium in the surface layer of the endothelium of skin blood vessels without accompanying water retention. The slope of the pressure-natriuretic relationship is less steep and shifts to the right in salt-sensitive individuals, and higher levels of blood pressure are required to increase sodium excretion and maintain sodium balance. Salt-sensitive individuals show sharp changes in blood pressure with acute or chronic salt deficiency or intake [2]. Also, the response of blood pressure to high sodium intake is individual due to the influence of genetic, hormonal, nervous and environmental factors, older age, obesity and black race. During salt sensitivity, there is an inadequate decrease in total peripheral resistance (TPR), which represents an acute (transient) change in blood pressure that disappears after a week. The long-term mechanism is greater sodium reabsorption in the PCT and an increase in the expression and activity of epithelial sodium channels (despite the reduction of aldosterone levels) [1]. Numerous factors have been proven that damage pressure natriuresis in the kidneys in the pathogenesis of salt-sensitive hypertension: autoimmune reactivity to the heat shock protein HSP70, SNPs in the sodium bicarbonate cotransporter gene SLC4A5 and SH2B adapter protein 3 genes, various inflammatory mediators such as gene-1 which activates recombination, interleukin (IL)-17A, interferon-gamma and IL-1β, low-potassium intake, dietary fructose, and increased reactive oxygen species (ROS) production. A low-potassium diet is associated with hypertension because potassium affects sodium reabsorption by modulating the activity of the sodium chloride cotransporter and epithelial sodium channels in the distal nephron [2]. Increased dietary intake of potassium leads to increased excretion of sodium in the distal tubules (K^+-induced diuresis) as a result of dephosphorylation of NCC mediated by phosphatases [27]. Dietary fructose supplementation before and during increased dietary salt intake promotes the development of salt-sensitive hypertension by modulating the activity and expression of the renal sodium transporter [2].

6. Pressure and natriuresis responses decrease with age

With age, there is a decrease in natriuresis, which causes an increase in blood pressure in people without chronic kidney disease. The drop in natriuretic response is not caused by reduced eGFR but by increased sympathetic tone, changes in renal blood vessels, a drop in ANP levels, and changes in the expression and activity of certain receptors. Changes in the renal microvasculature (reduced number of glomerular and peritubular capillaries) are associated with reduced autoregulation of renal perfusion pressure and increased sodium reabsorption. Despite the decrease in the renin-angiotensin-aldosterone system concentration with age, increased intrarenal formation of Ang II and increased sensitivity to aldosterone have been shown. There was also increased expression of renal AT 1 R and increased activity of medullary NKA, which directly stimulates Ang II in the proximal renal tubules. In the distal tubules, NCCs were more expressed in aged rats, and a possible enhancement of sodium retention *via* NCCs was suggested in human studies of hypertensive subjects because the thiazide diuretic effect increased with age. That is why previously, some guidelines for the treatment of hypertension suggested that salt restriction and diuretics are the most effective antihypertensive treatment measures in elderly people [3].

7. Conclusion

Pressure natriuresis is one of the fundamental and most important mechanisms of normal blood pressure regulation. A complex set of mechanisms is responsible for the proper regulation of pressure antidiuresis, and consequently, various imbalances of this network may lead to elevated blood pressure and hypertension. A good understanding of these mechanisms is crucial for an integrated understanding of whole blood pressure regulation and is also key for the future development of personalized and targeted treatment approaches.

Conflict of interest

The authors have no conflict of interest to declare.

Author details

Vedran Đambić[1] and Aleksandar Kibel[1,2,3*]

1 Department of Physiology and Immunology, Faculty of Medicine, J.J. Strossmayer University of Osijek, Osijek, Croatia

2 International Medical Center Priora, Čepin, Croatia

3 Department of Clinical Medicine, Faculty of Dental Medicine and Health, J.J. Strossmayer University of Osijek, Osijek, Croatia

*Address all correspondence to: aleksandar_mf@yahoo.com; aleksandar.kibel@priora.eu and aleksandar.kibel@mefos.hr

IntechOpen

References

[1] Díaz-Morales N, Baranda-Alonso EM, Martínez-Salgado C, López-Hernández FJ. Renal sympathetic activity: A key modulator of pressure natriuresis in hypertension. Biochemical Pharmacology. 2023;**208**:115386

[2] Baek EJ, Kim S. Current understanding of pressure Natriuresis. Electrolyte Blood Press. 2021;**19**(2):38-45

[3] Kim YG, Moon JY, Oh B, Chin HJ, Kim DK, Park JH, et al. Pressure-Natriuresis response is diminished in old age. Frontiers in Cardiovascular Medicine. 2022;**9**:840840

[4] Bernal A, Zafra MA, Simón MJ, Mahía J. Sodium homeostasis, a balance necessary for life. Nutrients. 2023;**15**(2):395

[5] Bulger DA, Griendling KK. Novel mechanism by which extracellular cyclic GMP induces Natriuresis. Circulation Research. 2023;**132**(9):1141-1143

[6] Parker MD, Myers EJ, Schelling JR. Na+-H+ exchanger-1 (NHE1) regulation in kidney proximal tubule. Cellular and Molecular Life Sciences. 2015;**72**(11):2061-2074

[7] Moreno E, Pacheco-Alvarez D, Chávez-Canales M, Elizalde S, Leyva-Ríos K, Gamba G. Structure-function relationships in the sodium chloride cotransporter. Frontiers in Physiology. 2023;**14**:1118706

[8] Snyder PM. The epithelial Na+ channel: Cell surface insertion and retrieval in Na+ homeostasis and hypertension. Endocrine Reviews. 2002;**23**(2):258-275

[9] Rout P, Jialal I. Hyperphosphatemia. In: StatPearls [Internet]. Treasure Island (FL): StatPearls Publishing; 2023. p. 2024

[10] Kemp BA, Howell NL, Gildea JJ, Hinkle JD, Shabanowitz J, Hunt DF, et al. Evidence that binding of cyclic GMP to the extracellular domain of NKA (sodium-potassium ATPase) mediates Natriuresis. Circulation Research. 2023;**132**(9):1127-1140

[11] Castrop H, Schießl IM. Physiology and pathophysiology of the renal Na-K-2Cl cotransporter (NKCC2). American Journal of Physiology. Renal Physiology. 2014;**307**(9):F991-F1002

[12] Sparks MA, Dilmen E, Ralph DL, Rianto F, Hoang TA, Hollis A, et al. Vascular control of kidney epithelial transporters. American Journal of Physiology. Renal Physiology. 2021;**320**(6):F1080-F1092

[13] Leite APO, Li XC, Nwia SM, Hassan R, Zhuo JL. Angiotensin II and AT1a receptors in the proximal tubules of the kidney: New roles in blood pressure control and hypertension. International Journal of Molecular Sciences. 2022;**23**(5):2402

[14] Carey RM, Siragy HM, Gildea JJ, Keller SR. Angiotensin Type-2 receptors: Transducers of Natriuresis in the renal proximal tubule. International Journal of Molecular Sciences. 2022;**23**(4):2317

[15] Mahía J, Bernal A, García Del Rio C, Puerto A. The natriuretic effect of oxytocin blocks medial Tuberomammillary polydipsia and polyuria in male rats. The European Journal of Neuroscience. 2009;**29**:1440-1446

[16] Culshaw G, Binnie D, Dhaun N, Hadoke P, Bailey M, Webb DJ. The acute pressure natriuresis response is suppressed by selective ETA receptor blockade. Clinical Science (London, England). 2021;**136**(1):15-28

[17] Soares AG, Contreras J, Mironova E, Archer CR, Stockand JD, Abd El-Aziz TM. P2Y2 receptor decreases blood pressure by inhibiting ENaC. JCI Insight. 2023;**8**(14):e167704

[18] Vendrov AE et al. Renal NOXA1/NOX1 signaling regulates epithelial sodium channel and sodium retention in angiotensin II-induced hypertension. Antioxidants & Redox Signaling. 2022;**36**(7-9):550-566

[19] Zeng C, Armando I, Yang J, Jose PA. Dopamine receptor D1R and D3R and GRK4 interaction in hypertension. The Yale Journal of Biology and Medicine. 2023;**96**(1):95-105

[20] Azzam O, Matthews VB, Schlaich MP. Interaction between sodium-glucose co-transporter 2 and the sympathetic nervous system. Current Opinion in Nephrology and Hypertension. 2022;**31**(2):135-141

[21] Heise T, Jordan J, Wanner C, Heer M, Macha S, Mattheus M, et al. Acute pharmacodynamic effects of empagliflozin with and without diuretic agents in patients with type 2 diabetes mellitus. Clinical Therapeutics. 2016;**38**:2248-2264

[22] Kumagai H, Oshima N, Matsuura T, Iigaya K, Imai M, Onimaru H, et al. Importance of rostral ventrolateral medulla neurons in determining efferent sympathetic nerve activity and blood pressure. Hypertension Research. 2012;**35**(2):132-141

[23] Frame AA, Nist KM, Kim K, Kuwabara JT, Wainford RD. Natriuresis during an acute intravenous sodium chloride infusion in conscious Sprague Dawley rats is mediated by a blood pressure-independent α1-adrenoceptor-mediated mechanism. Frontiers in Physiology. 2022;**12**:784957

[24] Genovesi S, Pieruzzi F, Wijnmaalen P, Centonza L, Golin R, Zanchetti A, et al. Renal afferents signaling diuretic activity in the cat. Circulation Research. 1993;**73**(5):906-913

[25] Wen Y, Crowley SD. Renal effects of cytokines in hypertension. Current Opinion in Nephrology and Hypertension. 2018;**27**(2):70-76

[26] Balasubbramanian D, Baranwal G, Clark MC, Goodlett BL, Mitchell BM, Rutkowski JM. Kidney-specific lymphangiogenesis increases sodium excretion and lowers blood pressure in mice. Journal of Hypertension. 2020;**38**(5):874-885

[27] Gritter M, Rotmans JI, Hoorn EJ. Role of dietary K+ in natriuresis, blood pressure reduction, cardiovascular protection, and Renoprotection. Hypertension. 2019;**73**(1):15-23

Chapter 3

Classification of Hemodynamics Using Ambulatory Blood Pressure Data

Margarita Voitikova and Raissa Khursa

Abstract

In medical practice, it is relevant to develop new methods for assessing the state of a patient's hemodynamics in everyday activities based on ambulatory blood pressure monitoring (ABPM) data. Of interest to the clinician is the analysis of ABPM using linear (regression and statistical) and nonlinear methods in both normal and pathological conditions. We present a new linear diagnostic tool and classification method in hemodynamics: regression modeling of ABPM to determine the hemodynamic phenotype in different categories of people. The linear regression of blood pressure parameters (LRBPP method) allows the differentiation of patients with dysfunctional diastolic and harmonic phenotypes in normotensive, hypotensive, and hypertensive individuals. Additionally, fractal analysis, one of the methods of nonlinear dynamics, has been used to assess the chaotic component of blood circulation. Thus, the value of the fractal dimension of ABPM time series, along with the application of the LRBPP method, can be used as a diagnostic criterion for assessing the state of hemodynamics and adaptation, as well as providing feedback for rapid and reliable correction of patient therapy.

Keywords: ambulatory blood pressure monitoring, hemodynamics, linear regression, fractal analysis, arterial hypertension, obstructive sleep apnea

1. Introduction

Arterial hypertension (AH) remains the most acute problem due to its ever-increasing prevalence and key role in the development of severe cardiovascular complications [1, 2]. Despite effective methods of AH treatment, the frequency of hypertension control is no more than 14% (according to the World Health Organization). The problem of poor hypertension control is often associated with a well-known issue in modern medicine—an insufficiently personalized approach to treatment: the absence of consideration for various concomitant diseases and cardiovascular risk factors, failure to assess the patient's adherence to drug therapy, and especially, failure to promote lifestyle modification.

As is well known, any chronic disease has a latent period of its development, so it can be expected that obvious hypertension is preceded by a period of hidden circulatory disorders, which dictates the necessity of adequate diagnostic methods.

At present, mathematical modeling and simulation of physiological systems are common features of biomedical research. The mathematical modeling of hemodynamics based on ambulatory blood pressure monitoring (ABPM) data offers numerous benefits, as it helps to understand principles, regulatory processes, and predict outcomes in the cardiovascular system [3]. Achievements in medical technologies and computer equipment significantly increase the potential of ABPM, determined by the methodology of medical signal analysis.

Hemodynamics can be described by a complex and nonlinear dynamic model that reproduces basic heart rhythms and regulatory processes, mean arterial pressure, systolic (SBP) and diastolic (DBP) blood pressure, the resistance of peripheral vessels, aortic elasticity, and the concentration of norepinephrine, among other factors [4]. The proposed integrative physiological model provides an adequate description of baroreflex and heart rhythm variability, short-term blood pressure variability, the spectral and statistical properties of heart rhythm, and other blood pressure parameters. However, researchers have had to resort to simplification in ABPM modeling due to the impossibility of accounting for all components of the integrative cardiovascular system and non-periodic fluctuations determined by the interaction of external and internal environments [5].

Earlier studies of the dynamics of 24-hour blood pressure (BP) time series [6–8] have shown the diagnostic potential of the linear regression of diastolic blood pressure (DBP) on systolic blood pressure (SBP) for the indirect determination of the rigidity of blood vessels (the so-called ambulatory arterial stiffness index—AASI), as regression coefficients are correlated with PWV.

According to Anokhin's theory of functional systems [9], the functioning of a system is characterized not only by its components, but also by the connections between them. If we consider BP as a functional system represented by components SBP, DBP, and pulse pressure PP (PP = SBP − DBP), then the relationships between them characterize this system. Specifically, considering SBP as an "input" and DBP as an "output," PP represents the system's "state" that determines its future behavior. Therefore, we used PP as an argument in the linear dependence of SBP and DBP on it, with the individual regression coefficients characterizing the hemodynamic features [10]. In this context, data mining algorithms [11], particularly Support Vector Machine (SVM), applied to the regression coefficients of BP parameters, are promising tools for transforming BP time series into new clinical information, including information on clinically latent circulatory problems [10, 12–16].

2. Materials and methods

The study was performed on 24-h ABPM data of the Belarus State Medical Universities of Minsk and Grodno (Belarus), 8 polyclinics (outpatient service), and four hospitals (inpatient service). ABPM were performed with an oscillometric device BPLab (Russia, https://bplab.ru) and CARDIAN MD (Belarus, https://cardian.by), which provided a measure of SBP and DBP every 15 min in daytime period, 30 min in night, and at least 24 hours of length. We also used MIMIC II Clinical Database [17], (https://physionet.org/content/mimic-ii/2.6.0/), which includes BP time series of patients with acute hypotension. We studied the distribution of phenotypes (see below) in different categories of patients: healthy patients and hypertensive ones, patients with coronary heart disease, stroke, and other diseases (more than 2.5 thousand people of different ages participated in the studies). Additionally, in normotensive healthy young adults, we examined the PWV and endothelium-dependent vasodilation by rheographic methods.

Because of the difference of the SBP and DBP values measured by different methods, the comparing of the BP data is incorrect. However, we have found that the regression modeling of the BP time series almost does not depend on the measurement method, therefore, comparative analysis can be performed for all available data. Furthermore, the removal of a few measurements or resampling of BP time series has very little effect on the regression coefficients. Artifacts were removed from all signals, after which we performed the linear regression of the BP data. This defined a vector of attributes with coordinates equal to the linear regression coefficients.

Before the regression modeling, the BP recordings were divided into three groups: arterial hypertensive (AH, a group of newly diagnosed non-treated AH), normotensive, and hypotensive groups.

3. Linear regression of BP parameters, LRBPP method

Systemic circulation is generated by the pressure difference between the aorta and the right atrium. Arterial BP varies between SBP and DBP during each heartbeat (cardio cycle) and correlates with left ventricular (LV) ejection, arterial stiffness, and pulse pressure PP. The last one is the result of the interaction between the contractile function of the heart and the "peripheral component"—primarily the vessels. This is why PP, as a pressure gradient, is an important differentiated characteristic of hemodynamics [12].

BP can be represented mathematically by a regression function of SBP on PP (method LRBPP, Linear Regression of BP Parameters [10, 12–19]). Based on this assumption, two regression coefficients {Q, a}, can be calculated according to the regression formulas: SBP = $Q + a$•PP (similarly, DBP = $Q + (a - 1)$•PP).

The angular coefficient a constitutes a variable component of BP since it specifies the proportion between the left the "peripheral component", primarily the vasculature. Coefficient Q is the static component of the blood flow and theoretically corresponds to the mean hemodynamic pressure MP. Assuming Q = MP, it is obvious that the known normal physiological ratio SBP > MP > DBP is possible only at $0 < a < 1$ (harmonious H-phenotype, **Figure 1**). Thus, harmonic phenotype of blood circulation corresponds to the normal cardiovascular interaction, in which the patient's heart performs the majority of work in the blood circulation compared with the vessels. It should be noted that H-phenotype can be accompanied by different values of Q. Our studies have shown that the prevalence of the H-phenotype is 65–75% of healthy normotensive young people (Section 6.1).

The value $a > 1$ and SBP > DBP > Q in the equation DBP = $Q + (a - 1)$. PP indicates a reverse component for diastolic pressure (diastolic dysfunction circulation), **Figure 2**. This trend is characteristic of circulation disorders where blood circulation is primarily maintained by the myocardium due to arterial stiffness and/or insufficient participation of the peripheral component (Section 6.2).

If $a < 0$, then Q > SBP > DBP, S-phenotype (systolic dysfunctional circulation) is recognized, which suggests an abnormally high role of the peripheral component in maintaining the circulation.

According to our observations, many people have dysfunctional phenotypes. In particular, D-phenotype present in young patients, especially those with insufficient

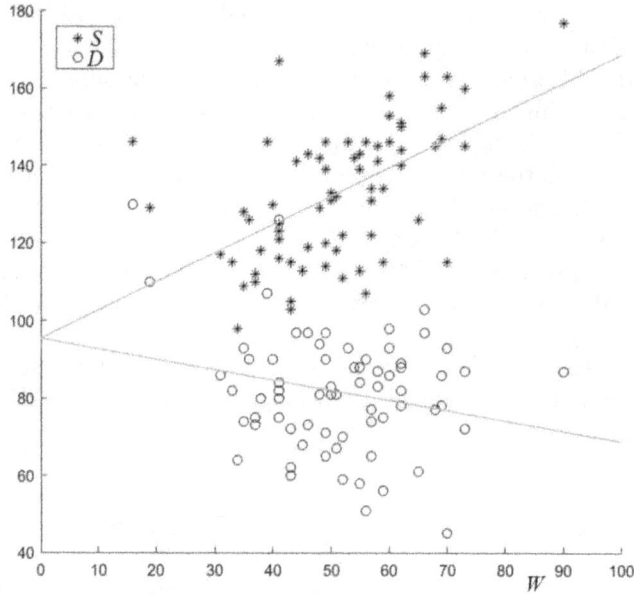

Figure 1.
Harmonic phenotype of hemodynamics: regression of systolic and diastolic pressure on pulse pressure and regression line [13].

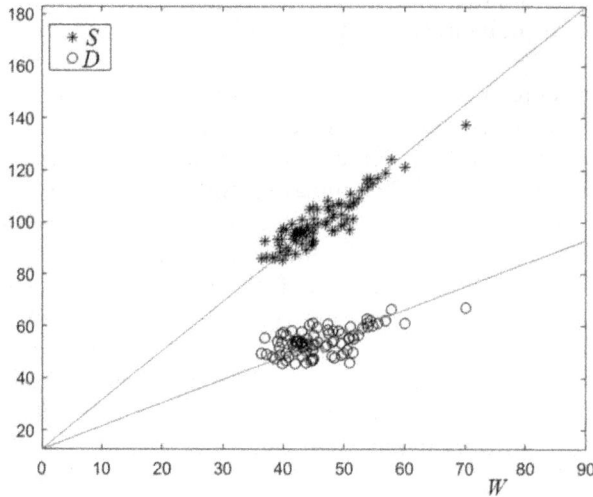

Figure 2.
Diastolic phenotype of hemodynamics: regression of systolic and diastolic pressure on pulse pressure and regression line [13].

physical activity (~8–20%) and in hypertensive patients (≥40%). The prevalence of D-phenotype increases with age in the general population. The S-phenotype is very rare in general population (~1.5–3.5%), more common in young athletes (~5–6%), and very rare in older people and hypertensive patients (~0.5–1.5%).

The values of the coefficients {Q, a} and the Pearson correlation coefficient r_{SD} can be determined by the following mathematical expression (where N is the number of measurements):

$$a = \frac{N\Sigma(SBP \cdot PP) - \Sigma SBP \cdot \Sigma PP}{N\Sigma PP^2 - (\Sigma PP)^2}, Q = mean(SBP) - a \cdot mean(PP). \tag{1}$$

As can be seen, the regression coefficients are related to the standard deviations of SBP and DBP by a simple relation:

$$a = \frac{k_1 - k_3}{k_1 - 2k_3 + k_2}, Q = (1-a)\sqrt{\frac{\Sigma SBP^2 - k_1}{N}} + a\sqrt{\frac{\Sigma DBP^2 - k_2}{N}},$$

$$r_{SD} = \frac{k_3}{\sqrt{k_1 k_2}}, k_1 = (N-1) \cdot std(SBP)^2, k_2 = (N-1) \cdot std(DBP)^2,$$

$$k_3 = \Sigma(SBP \cdot DBP) - \sqrt{(\Sigma SBP^2 - k_1) \cdot (\Sigma DBP^2 - k_2)} \tag{2}$$

It can be shown in Eq. (2), that the changes in the hemodynamic phenotype occur when k_1–k_3 = 0 for a = 0 (dysfunctional systolic phenotype of hemodynamic is replaced by a harmonic phenotype) and k_2–k_3 = 0 for a = 1 (harmonic phenotype of hemodynamics is replaced by dysfunctional diastolic phenotype).

Obviously, the main factors that can adversely affect the accuracy and significance of the {Q, a} are the nonstationarity and/or short length of BP recordings, the physiological and technical artifacts, noise, etc.

4. Classification of ABPM samples

The coefficients of linear regression of ABPM can be plotted in the parametric plane {Q, a}, hereinafter referred to as the diagnostic nomogram for hemodynamic classification (**Figures 3** and **4**).

The diagnostic nomogram was created with application of discriminative SVM classifier [11]. The goal of *SVM* is to find the optimal hyperplane that maximizes the margin between some classes. Since each BP signal is represented as a feature vector x = {Q, a} in feature space and belongs to one of the three classes (*Hypotension-Normotension-Hypertension*), maximizing the margin leads to more reliable classification, in our case—the phenotype of hemodynamics. Moreover, the *SVM* classifier can provide high-quality separation of hemodynamic phenotypes using only a few parameters of BP time series, as it leverages the vector model representation of the BP signal, regardless of arbitrary sampling frequency, duration, or missing data.

Figure 3 shows two-dimensional diagnostic nomogram of the linear regression coefficients {Q, a} for 24-hour ABPM data. Triangles represent patients with hypertension, asterisks indicate hypotension, and circles denote normotensive patients with harmonic (transparent circles) and diastolic hemodynamics (semi-transparent). Due to circadian rhythms, the patient's blood flow varies during the day and night periods.

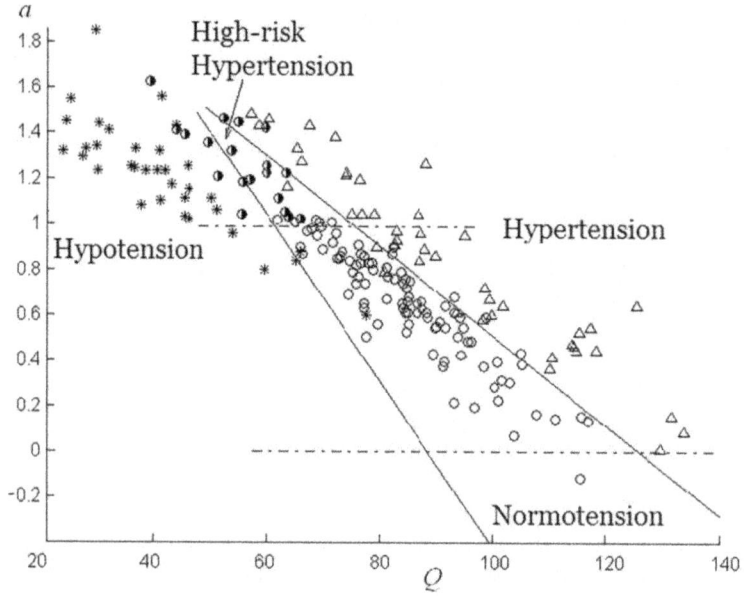

Figure 3.
Diagnostic nomogram {Q, a}. Classification of 24-h BP data [13].

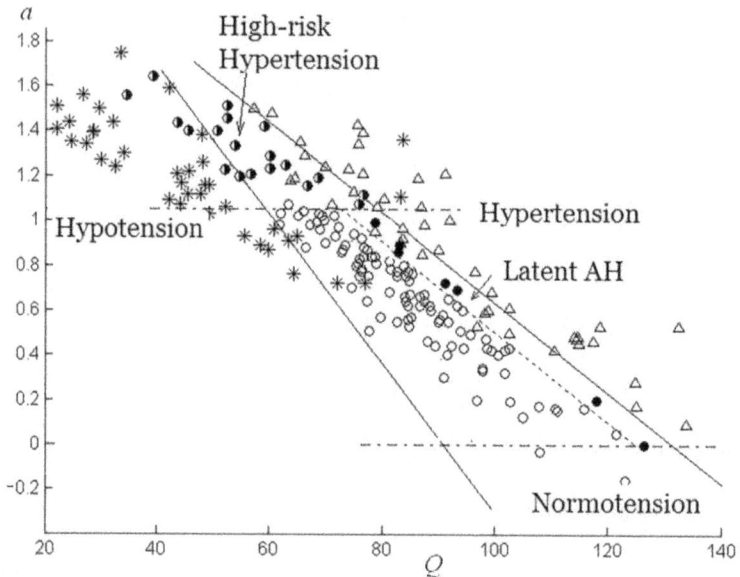

Figure 4.
Diagnostic nomogram {Q, a}. Classification of daytime BP data [13].

Therefore, we analyzed BP time series separately for the day and the 24-hour period.
Figure 4 shows the SVM classification with the linear separation functions for daytime
measurements of BP.

5. Summary of hemodynamic classification method

According to the proposed diagnostic method, each BP recording of the tested data is represented as a point on the nomogram belonging to a certain area: AH, hypotension, or normotension. As a result, up to 9 hemodynamic classes can be diagnosed on 24-h nomogram, **Figure 5**: in patients with normal BP level (diastolic D2-class, harmonic H2-class), in hypertensive patients (diastolic D3-class, harmonic H3-class), or in hypotensive classes (D1-class and H1-class in **Figure 5**). Thus, the functional status of harmonious blood circulation, adequate to the normotension and normal physiology of the heart/vessels interaction, is described by separating lines for 24-hour BP recordings: $-0.037Q + 3.28 < a < -0.02Q + 2.52$ and $0 < a < 1$ (**Figure 5**). The location of linear regression coefficients outside these thresholds indicates a pathological change in the hemodynamics, including hypertension and hypotension, which are accompanied by both normal and disproportionate contribution of the heart and vessels to the blood circulation (dysfunctional hemodynamics).

A nomogram implemented for the daytime period of the ABPM defined 10 hemo-dynamic classes (**Figure 6**). Modeling only the daytime ABPM data, the thresholds for normotension status are: $-0.03Q + 3.03 < a < -0.02Q + 2.52$ and $0 < a < 1$.

Based on the proposed classification, latent hemodynamic disturbances in normotensive patients are associated with dysfunctional classes (diastolic D2- or systolic - S2-class). Hypertensive patients are represented by two classes, D3 and H3, with a dysfunctional diastolic and harmonic phenotype of the blood circulation. Among latent hemodynamic disturbances in the cohort of normotensive patients, we highlight H0-class (so-called Quasi-hypertension, **Figure 6**) as prehypertension status because the hemodynamics of patients in the H0-class are similar to patients

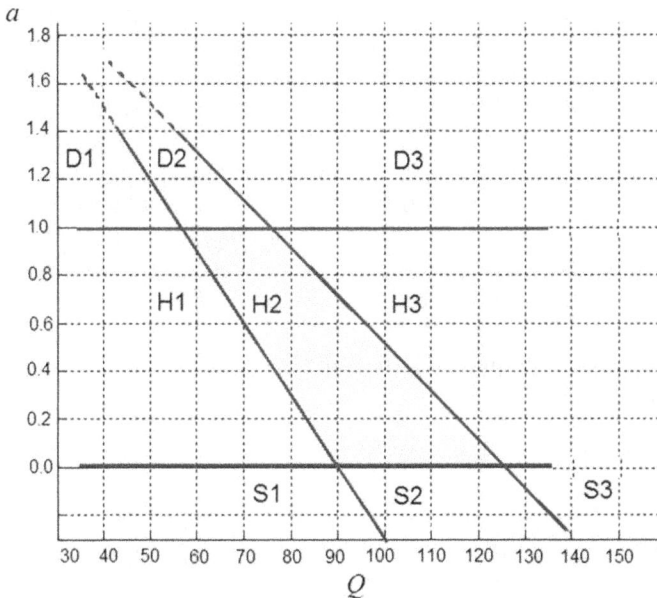

Figure 5.
Diagnostic nomogram for 24-hour ABPM [13].

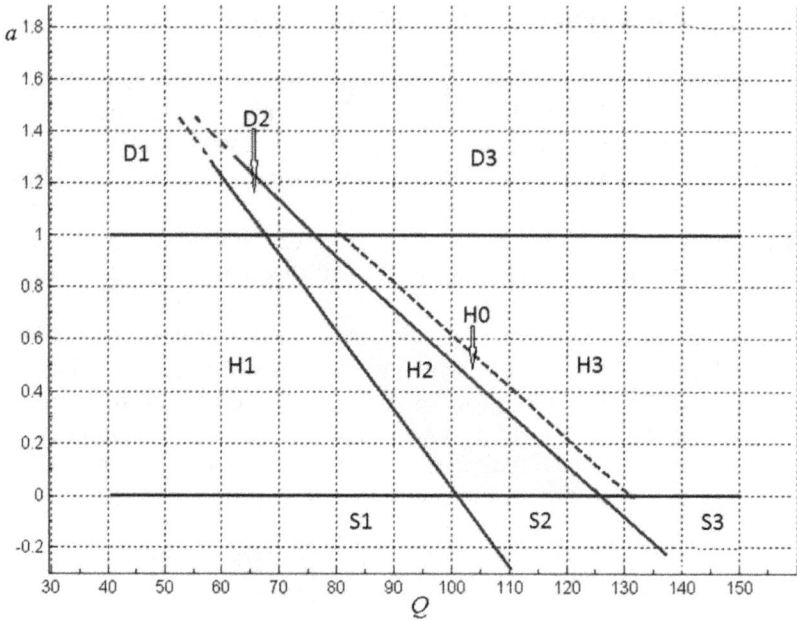

Figure 6.
Diagnostic nomogram for daytime ABPM [13].

with hypertension before treatment (H3-class) [12–16]. In other words, H0-class is the area on daytime nomogram, where the sets of BP parameters of hypertensive and normotensive individuals overlap. Patients in the H0-class can be classified as the normotensive or hypertensive on the 24-hour nomogram, depending on BP at night. The thresholds of parameters for daytime ABPM recordings for the H0-class are: $-0.02Q + 2.52 < a < -0.02Q + 2.62$ and $0 < a < 1$ (**Figure 6**).

In the nomogram, ABPM of hypotensive patients is represented by D1- and H1-class areas with a dysfunctional diastolic and harmonic phenotype of blood circulation. For example, ABPM data of patients with secondary hypotension due to severe diseases (heart attack, stroke, bleeding, etc., [17]) have $\{Q, a\}$ located in D1-class area. These patients are characterized by diastolic circulatory dysfunction and low mean pressure ($a > 1$, $Q < 70$).

Thus, the nomogram allows for the diagnosis of the following hemodynamic classes:

- Hypotensive: harmonious (H1), diastolic dysfunctional (D1), systolic dysfunctional (S1);

- Normotensive: harmonious (H2), diastolic dysfunctional (D2), systolic dysfunctional (S2);

- Hypertensive: harmonious (H3), diastolic dysfunctional (D3), systolic dysfunctional (S3); quasi-hypertension (H0).

The following hemodynamic classes have clinical significance, as we established: "Hypotensive Diastolic"—D1, "Normotensive Diastolic"—D2, "Hypertensive Diastolic"—D3, "Normotensive Harmonic"—H2, "Hypertensive Harmonic"—H3,

"Normotensive Systolic"—S2. It should be noted that no actual ABPM samples of classes: "Hypotensive Harmonic"—H1; "Hypotensive, Hypertensive Systolic"—S1, S3. According to our observations, the "Normotensive Systolic" S2 class is inherent in athletes ("peripheral heart" phenomenon).

Now consider the ability of the nomogram to retrace changes in hemodynamics of a patient due to antihypertensive therapy. Consider the simultaneous increase or decrease of the systolic SBP and diastolic DBP pressure of the patient by Δ mmHg. As can be seen in Eqs. (1) and (2), such an increase or decrease in BP level is equivalent to a shift to the right or left on the nomogram, when $Q_{\pm\Delta} = Q \pm \Delta$, $a_{\pm\Delta} = a$.

In other words, changing the diastolic phenotype of hemodynamics to the harmonious phenotype (i.e. H3 ← D3 or H2 ← D2) is impossible by merely decreasing systolic or/and diastolic BP, which is equivalent to the "horizontal" displacement on the nomogram. A similar situation is observed for the treatment of hypotensive patients, where the therapeutic effect is aimed at increasing the BP level (i.e. D2 ← D1).

6. Clinical application of the diagnostic nomogram and regression modeling of ABPM

For more than 20 years, we have been studying phenotypes and classes by linear regression of ABPM in different categories of patients, including healthy individuals. Regression modeling represents the simplest statistical model of the patient's blood circulation, as well as the dynamic changes in BP due to the combined efforts of the heart and the "peripheral" component (vessels, muscles). The values of the regression coefficients $\{Q, a\}$ show the relationships between the parameters of BP in a particular patient (their strength and direction), Eq. (1). **Figure 7** shows the scheme for hemodynamic phenotypes and classes. LRBPP of ABPM is included in the software for long-term ECG and BP monitoring systems CARDIAN-MD (Cardian, Belarus, https://cardian.by) [18]. A computing unit automatically displays the individual coefficients of regressions, the diagnostic nomograms for three observation periods, and a conclusion about the hemodynamic class.

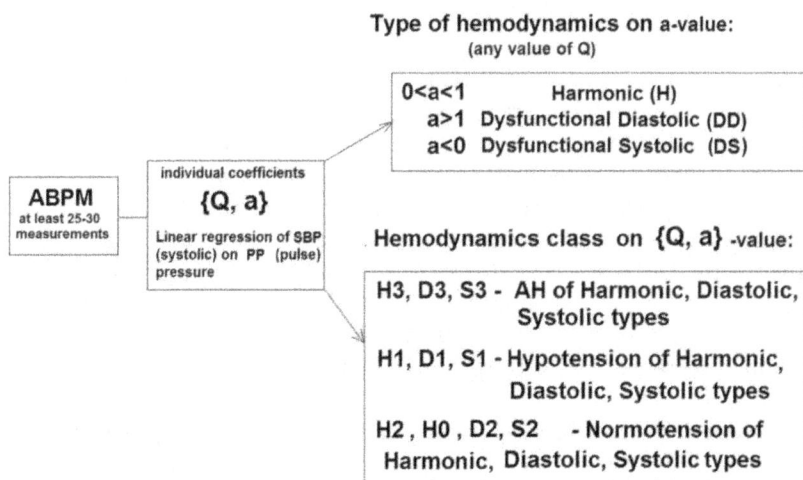

Figure 7.
Hemodynamic phenotypes and classes [10].

In addition, we defined other hemodynamic parameters for patients: PWV along the carotid-radial pathway (PWV) and endothelium-dependent vasodilation (EDVD) by rheographic methods and conventional ABPM parameters.

6.1 The hemodynamic phenotypes in population. Pathological phenotypes in young normotensive people

The distribution of the hemodynamic phenotypes in the population depends on the age and health status of patients and does not differ significantly between men and women. In particular, the proportion of the harmonic phenotype (H) decreases with age due to vascular stiffness, AH in anamnesis, and associated cardiovascular pathology. It should be noted that S-phenotype (dysfunctional systolic phenotype, "peripheral heart" model) is very rare in the population, especially in those with AH [10]. Among healthy young people with different levels of physical state (students, aged 22.8 ± 0.56 years), H-phenotype is presented in 63.7–72%, D-phenotype—15.9–18.3%, S-phenotype—3.8–6.1%. Among outpatients with AH of middle and older age, the D-phenotype was observed in 40.8–46.3%, H-phenotype—in 53.1–58.1%, and S-phenotype—0.6–1.1%.

The results of our studies have shown that among healthy young people only 58.7% had optimally normal blood circulation (H2-class), the rest had pathological phenotypes: D-phenotype (D1–D3 classes), S-phenotype (S2 and S3 classes), as well as hypertensive H-phenotype (H3-class and borderline H0-class). We also analyzed the pulse wave velocity (PWV) along the carotid-radial pathway and endothelium-dependent vasodilation (EDVD) by rheographic methods using digital computer interpretive impedance cardiograph INTECARD-M (http://intecard.by), depending on the phenotype [10]. In normotensive young people with the D-phenotype, PWV was statistically higher than in H-phenotype (11.4 (8.1–13.7) and 8.1 (7.0–9.5) resp., $p < 0.05$) and did not differ from hypertensive patients (11.4 (8.0–13.5), $p > 0.05$). In hypertensive patients, there were no differences in PWV between H- and D-phenotypes. Moderate and severe EDVD disorders were observed in normotensive individuals of the D-phenotype in 62.5%; and in H-phenotype individuals—21.6%. Among patients with AH, these disorders were present in 69.6% and 56.2%, respectively. Thus, the similarity of the functional state of blood vessels in healthy individuals of the D-phenotype and hypertensive patients became obvious.

Moreover, compared with the H2-class, the patients with the D-phenotype had significantly higher diastolic pressure during the daytime and night periods ($p < 0.05$).

Interesting conclusions can be made about the effect of physical activity on the hemodynamic phenotype. The D-phenotype can be changed to H-phenotype (harmonic phenotype) in young people due to lifestyle changes (e.g. moderate physical fitness), as evidenced by a prospective observation using bicyclergometry (BET, **Figure 8**).

In other words, our research confirms the pathological nature of dysfunctional phenotypes (in particular, D-phenotype) and the hypertensive classes of H-phenotype (H0-class and H3-class), which indicates the need for further monitoring and detailed examination of these patients as the group of increased risk of developing AH.

6.2 Hemodynamic phenotypes in hypertensive patients during treatment

The study involved 267 outpatients with a verified AH diagnosis, including the comorbidity with chronic ischemic heart disease (CIHD) in some of them. All patients had a disease duration of 3–12 years and received treatment by antihypertensive drugs:

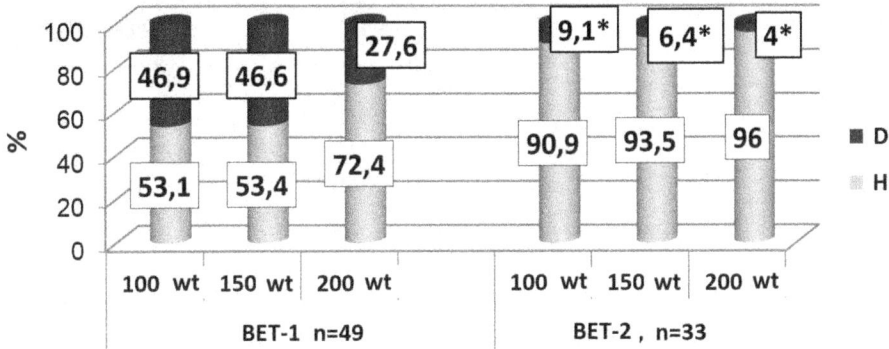

Figure 8.
*Distribution of phenotypes at the bicycle ergometric test: BET-1 (at the beginning) and BET-2 (after 6 months of regular physical activity) [10]. *—p < 0.05.*

angiotensin-converting enzyme inhibitors (ACEI) or angiotensin-II receptor blockers (ARB), thiazide-like diuretics (TLD), beta-blockers (BB), calcium channel blockers (CCB). In 175 patients from the observation group, the quality of life (QL) was determined according to the RAND-36 general questionnaire, validated and adapted to the Republic of Belarus. We analyzed clinical and demographic features, ongoing treatment, the achieving of target BP and the QL depending on the patient's hemodynamic phenotype. The patients with AH grade 2 predominated in the group—55.6%; the majority of patients in the group belonged to the category of high and very high cardiovascular risk—74.9%. Additionally, 43.1% had CIHD, including rhythm disturbances (mainly extrasystole) in 9.4%, myocardial infarction in anamnesis in 7.1%; acute cerebrovascular accident in anamnesis—2.6%, diabetes mellitus type 2—5.6%.

The distribution of hemodynamic phenotypes was as follows: H-phenotype—58.1% (155 persons), D—40.8% (109), S—1.1% (3). According to clinical characteristics, patients with the D-phenotype were statistically significantly different from those with the H-phenotype in a larger proportion of individuals with AH grade 3 (33.0% and 15.5%, respectively), and the number of patients, who reached the BP treatment target, 38.5% and 54.8%, respectively (p < 0.05) without gender differences. Additionally, among 84 patients with resistant hypertension, persons of the D-phenotype predominated significantly—61.9% (52 persons) compared with patients with the H-phenotype—38.1% (32 persons). This group of patients with the D-phenotype showed the worst efficacy of antihypertensive drug therapy compared with other groups of outpatients with hypertension.

In addition, we analyzed the probability of achieving the BP treatment target in patients with H- and D-phenotype depending on the drugs used from different pharmacological groups (monotherapy or in combination). It was found that the proportion of people with the D-phenotype who achieved the BP treatment target is less than those with the H-phenotype for any group of drugs used (**Table 1**) [10]. In patients with H-phenotype and concomitant CIHD, the effectiveness of achieving the BP target was also less than in its absence. Additionally, for the H-phenotype, the antihypertensive drugs BB and CCB showed the highest efficiency in achieving the BP target (75.7% (28 people) and 72.7% (8 people), respectively).

Thus, the achievement of the BP target in the D-phenotype did not depend on the number of antihypertensive drugs used, while in the H-phenotype, treatment with 1–2 drugs was more effective.

Antihypertensive drugs	Disease	H-phenotype		D-phenotype	
		n	BP treatment target, %	n	BP treatment target, %
ACEI/ARB, n = 215	AH and CIHD	62	45.2 (28)	43	30.2 (13)
	AH	54	61.1 (33)	53	42.3 (24)
	All	**116**	**52.6 (61)**	**96**	**39.5 (38)**[*]
BB, n = 106	AH and CIHD	26	57.5 (15)	23	30.4 (7)
	AH	37	75.7 (28)	19	57.9 (11)
	All	**63**	**68.2 (43)**	**42**	**45.2 (19)**[*]
CCB, n = 78	AH and CIHD	33	39.4 (13)	22	22.7 (5)
	AH	11	72.7 (8)	10	30.0 (3)
	All	**44**	**47.7 (21)**	**32**	**31.2 (10)**
TLD, n = 121	AH and CIHD	47	53.2 (25)	24	25.0 (6)[*]
	AH	23	56.5 (13)	25	40.0 (10)
	All	**69**	**55.1 (38)**	**49**	**32.6 (16)**[*]

[*]—p < 0.05 in H-phenotype; n—number of patients.

Table 1.
Achieving the BP treatment target in patients with hemodynamic H- and D-phenotype using the antihypertensive drugs [10].

The QL of patients with AH (regardless of phenotype) depended on age: it was worse mainly in terms of the physical component of health, in men after 45 years and in women after 54–55 years. The achievement of the BP treatment target for all phenotypes had a significant impact on QL. In individuals with the D-phenotype, if the BP treatment target was not achieved, QL was significantly worse across most scales, the total physical component, and the overall level of QL. In contrast, in persons with the H-phenotype, the impact was limited to the physical components of PF, RP, and the total physical component (**Table 2**).

Thus, any group of antihypertensive drugs, as well as any number of prescribed drugs from different groups, shows a low efficiency in achieving the BP treatment target in patients with the D-phenotype. As the intensification of drug treatment further reduces the QL, the treatment of hypertensive patients with the D-phenotype should initially be complex, with the use of additional therapeutic measures: non-drug methods and adjuvant means. First of all, it is necessary to modify the lifestyle with an increase in physical activity and individually selected therapeutic exercise, which follows from the essence of this phenotype (it theoretically assumes a "passive periphery" and, as shown above in Chapter 6.1, can change to a harmonic phenotype). Medicines that affect vascular rigidity, in particular vitamin D, can also be useful [19].

6.3 Hemodynamic phenotypes in obstructive sleep apnea

One of the clinical applications of the nomogram is the ability to retrace changes in hemodynamics of the patient due to antihypertensive therapy and continuous positive airway pressure therapy (CPAP). This is a critical area of research, as both hypertension and obstructive sleep apnea syndrome (OSA) are prevalent conditions that can significantly impact cardiovascular health.

QL, scales	Target BP reached			Target BP not reached		
	group	H, n = 47	D, n = 30	group	H, n = 24	D, n = 33
PF	70.0 (50.0–90.0)	75.0 (45.0–90.0)	67.5 (50.0–85.0)	45.0 (25.0–60.0)**	50.0 (32.5–72.5)*	45.0 (20.0–55.0)*
RP	66.6 (25.0–100)	60.0 (25.0–100)	70.8 (25.0–100.0)	25.0 (0.0–100.0)**	45.0 (0.0–87.5)	25.0 (0.0–100)*
BP	67.5 (55.0–90.0)	67.5 (55.0–87.5)	67.5 (55.0–90.0)	65.0 (45.0–77.5)**	57.5 (45.0–67.5)*	67.5 (45.0–80.0)
RE	66.6 (33.0–100)	66.0 (33.3–100)	66.0 (33.3–100.0)	66.6 (0.0–100.0)	66.0 (33.0–100)	33.3 (0.0–100.0)
EF	55.0 ± 2.23	54.9 ± 3.00	55.2 ± 3.36	47.6 ± 2.81**	50.8 ± 3.99	45.3 ± 3.89
EW	64.0 (52.0–72.0)	64.0 (52.0–72.0)	64.0 (52.0–75.0)	56.0** (44.0–65.0)	56.0 (48.0–64.5)	52.0 (44.0–68.0)*
SF	62.5 (50.0–87.5)	75.0 (50.0–87.5)	62.5 (62.5–87.5)	62.5 (50.0–87.5)	62.5 (50.0–81.3)	62.5 (50.0–87.5)
GH	47.1 ± 2.01	46.3 ± 3.00	48.5 ± 2.88	36.5 ± 2.68	39.4 ± 4.00	34.4 ± 3.61*
HC	50.0 (50.0–50.0)	50.0 (50.0–50.0)	50.0 (50.0–50.0)	50.0 (0.0–50.0)**	50.0 (25.0–50.0)	50.0 (0.0–50.0)*
Physical comp.	66.7 (46.7–86.7)	66.7 (45.8–88.3)	65.8 (46.7–85.0)	45.8 (30.8–70.8)**	46.3 (31.7–75.8)*	45.8 (28.3–68.3)*
Psych. comp.	62.9 (48.3–75.0)	62.9 (48.4–77.7)	63.6 (49.1–71.3)	54.7 (35.7–68.0)**	59.1 (41.5–70.3)	44.1 (32.3–68.0)
Social. comp.	58.8 (47.5–72.5)	61.3 (47.5–73.8)	57.6 (47.5–72.5)	50.0 (36.3–63.8)**	51.3 (43.8–64.4)	50.0 (32.3–63.8)
Total score QL	62.8 (48.5–76.4)	62.8 (48.5–76.5)	61.3 (48.3–74.9)	48.3 (37.4–65.8)**	51.4 (42.7–70.4)	46.3 (35.9–64.8)*

*Differences between those who achieved and did not achieve the target BP in the same phenotype, p < 0.05.
**Differences between those who achieved and did not achieve the target BP in the all group, p < 0.05.

Table 2.
Quality of life and achievement of BP target in the treatment of patients with hemodynamic H- and D-phenotype; Me (Q25–Q75) or M ± m [10].

Our previous study [20] aimed to understand how effective CPAP therapy is in modulating BP among hypertensive patients with OSA and to classify responses for potential therapeutic implications. The study included 33 patients with hypertension and moderate to severe OSA. All patients underwent ABPM twice: at baseline and after a week of CPAP. The phenotypes were determined by employing regression analyses during the day, night, and over the entire 24-hour period. CPAP performance was assessed as an additional 5% nocturnal reduction in BP compared with baseline ABPM. Using this criterion, patients were further classified as responders (who achieved this target) and non-responders.

All patients received antihypertensive treatment, and the diagnosis of OSA was made based on sleep polygraphy data and the respiratory event index during the month prior to the ABPM study. Differences in responder and non-responder groups were analyzed retrospectively to identify associations between baseline hemodynamic phenotype and CPAP therapy efficacy.

The statistical analysis of the ABPM data showed that none of the patients had a normal 24-hour ABPM profile with a 10–20% decrease in BP at night. The

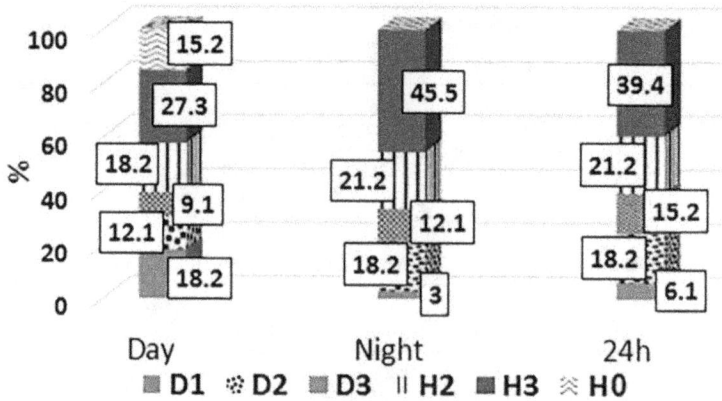

Figure 9.
Frequency of the hemodynamic classes for observation periods (daytime, nighttime, 24-hour), % [20].

hemodynamic classes for these patients are shown in **Figure 9**. Only 18.2% of patients could be assigned to the hemodynamic H2-class during the daytime period, despite combined antihypertensive therapy. Most patients were classified into the hemodynamic H3-class, including the nocturnal and 24-hour periods, confirming inadequate BP control in these patients.

The D1-class was diagnosed in 18.2% of patients during the daytime period. This class has a high risk of acute hypotensive episodes. Additionally, based on the daily nomogram, the hemodynamics of responders can be classified as H3-class, in contrast to the group of non-responders: 53.3% and 5.6%, respectively (**Figure 10**).

Only 21.2% of hypertensive patients with OSA who received complex antihypertensive therapy belonged to the class of optimal hemodynamics (H2-class), and most of the remaining patients had hemodynamics of the H3-class (39.4%) or diastolic dysfunctional D3-class (15.2%).

Non-responders demonstrated a phenomenon of phenotype transformation at nighttime, especially into classes H3 and D2 from other classes, versus responders

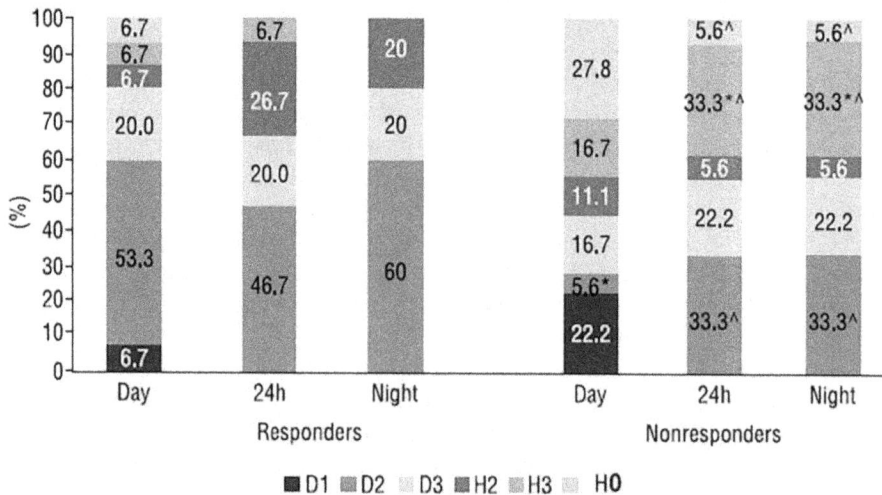

Figure 10.
Distribution of hemodynamic classes (frequency, %) [20]. ^p < 0.05.

(p < 0.05), and high variability of classes between observation periods. At night, the number of persons with H3-class (harmonious hypertensive hemodynamics) increased significantly from 5.6% to 33.3% (p = 0.005), indicating a negative hemodynamic tendency. However, at night, the number of persons with D1-class decreased compared to the daytime (p = 0.003), leading to an increase in the number of persons with D2-class (**Figure 9**). We assess such hemodynamics as positive, since the D1 class is dangerous due to acute hypotensive episodes, while the D2 class determines normotensive hemodynamics, although of a dysfunctional phenotype.

The differences between class H3 frequency in responders and non-responders allowed us to assess the probability of a positive response to CPAP (improvement in the diurnal index) in patients with this hemodynamic class during the daytime ABPM period: OR = 3.1 (CI95% 1.6–5.9), F = 0.3; p = 0.003. This means that patients with hemodynamic class H3 have a better treatment outcome with CPAP.

However, some non-responders also had positive results from CPAP, which included the transformation of D1-class during the daytime period into better hemodynamic classes at night and over 24 hours, first into D2-class. The difference in diurnal hemodynamics between non-responders and responders was significant: χ_{2MN} = 12.1, p < 0.001.

6.4 Hemodynamic phenotypes in chronic kidney disease patients

Chronic kidney disease (CKD) is characterized by various risk factors for the development of cardiovascular diseases (CVD), including vascular remodeling and hemodynamic disturbances.

While the progression of CKD involves numerous pathophysiological pathways, the activation of the sympathetic nervous system plays a key role in the development of CKD, its progression, arterial stiffening, and predicted CV mortality in patients with end-stage renal disease. Consequently, patients at all stages of CKD are at a higher risk of CV diseases compared to the general population and patients with hypertension and preserved kidney function.

The aim of the study [3] carried out at the University Clinical Centre in Gdansk (2019–2021) was to determine hemodynamic phenotypes based on linear regression of ABPM in stage G3–G4 CKD patients at very high CV risk. About 24-hour ambulatory BP monitoring (ABPM), carotid-femoral PWV, and central BP were obtained from 52 patients (aged 60 ± 11 years, 40% males, BMI 30 ± 6 kg/m^2) with stage 3–4 CKD (eGFR 44 ± 12 mL/min/1.73 m^2).

We performed regression modeling of ABPM data to determine the hemodynamic phenotypes of patients. Coexisting hypertension was present in 45 (86%) patients, out of whom 33 (73%) had controlled BP. About 26 patients demonstrated the harmonious (H) phenotype, and 26 patients demonstrated the diastolic dysfunctional (D) phenotype. eGFR was not significantly different between both phenotypes. Compared to the H-phenotype, patients with the D-phenotype were older (57 ± 11 vs. 63 ± 10 years, p = 0.04), had higher PWV (8.2 [7.3–10.3] vs. 9.7 [8.3–10.9] m/s, p = 0.02), ambulatory arterial stiffness index (AASI) (0.31 ± 0.1 vs. 0.40 ± 0.1, p = 0.02), systolic BP (128 [122–130] vs. 137 [130–150] mm Hg, p = 0.001), and systolic BP variability (BPV) (11.7 ± 2.3 vs. 15.7 ± 3.4 mm Hg, p < 0.0001). Thus, one in two patients without clinically overt cardiovascular disease (CV) with stage G3–G4 CKD demonstrates an unfavorable hemodynamic D-phenotype associated with higher PWV, AASI, systolic BP, and systolic BPV.

The linear regression model (LRBPP model) may be useful in detecting latent abnormalities in patients with controlled BP. Determining the hemodynamic phenotype by LRBPP from 24-hour ABPM seems to be an easily available, non-invasive tool to potentially identify individuals predisposed to CV complications.

7. Fractality of ABPM time series

BP and heart rate are not constant over any time period but fluctuate in a complex manner. This behavior determines the self-organization and adaptation of all living organisms [21–23]. In other words, irregularity, unpredictability, and randomness are reliable characteristics of health, and a decrease in variability, loss of randomness, as well as the emergence of pronounced periodicity, serve as signs of (existing or progressive) pathology in various diseases. In this context, fractal analysis of ABPM can be very effective for understanding the complexity of the cardiac system, as data exhibit scale-invariant features and self-similarity (correlation, memory).

The aims of this study [24] were to compare the results of LRBPP and fractal analyses of ABPM (about 150 samples of daytime ABPM from healthy volunteers, hypo- and hypertensive patients, Section 2) and to determine the prognostic potential of the fractal dimension (FD). The choice of the daytime period for the ABPM time series was due to the exclusion of daytime/nighttime fluctuations in BP levels.

Usually, the concept of fractality as a model is used if a real physiological object with non-deterministic behavior cannot be represented by classical models (trend, linear regression, etc.), which assume that the future is quite deterministic. Fractal analysis of any physiological signals cannot be performed without an a priori model that has essential features of the physiological process. The fractional Brownian motion (fBm) [25, 26] is the main fractal model for human biosignals, including ABPM time series. The self-similarity parameter of fBm is the Hurst exponent (H) in the range [0, 1]. It is a cardinal measure of the stochastic process: if $0.5 < H < 1$—the process has long-range correlation and pronounced trends; $H = 0.5$—the process is a random uncorrelated Wiener process (classical Brownian motion); $0 < H < 0.5$ indicates an anti-correlated or antipersistent fBm process.

Let us consider a time series of ABPM, which presumably consists of quasi-periodic and random oscillations, as well as fractal structures. In particular, ABPM is a discrete-time series of systolic and diastolic BP as a function of measurement time: SBP = {s1, s2, ..., sN} and DBP = {d1, d2, ..., dN} with the amplitude determined for the current measurement index. Since the index increases linearly from 1 to N (amplitude is the fractal variable), it is assumed that SBP and DBP are one-dimensional fractal sets, the FD of which is within [1, 2], and the Hurst exponent is given by the relation: $H = 2 - FD$ [25, 26].

The main problem of reliable FD estimation is the short duration of ABPM series because a short signal becomes more similar to a random dataset, and the uncertainty of FD increases. Therefore, we considered the methods suitable for non-stationary or short ABPM time series: the Higuchi algorithm and the least coverage method [5, 25].

In the first stage, the LRBPP method was used on the daytime ABPM data of 57 healthy volunteers (normotensive harmonic H2-class), 47 hypertensive patients (patients represented by two classes: hypertensive harmonic H3-class and hypertensive diastolic D3-class), and 25 patients with secondary hypotension and severe cardiovascular disease (hypotensive diastolic D1-class). In the second stage, the

Fractal Dimension

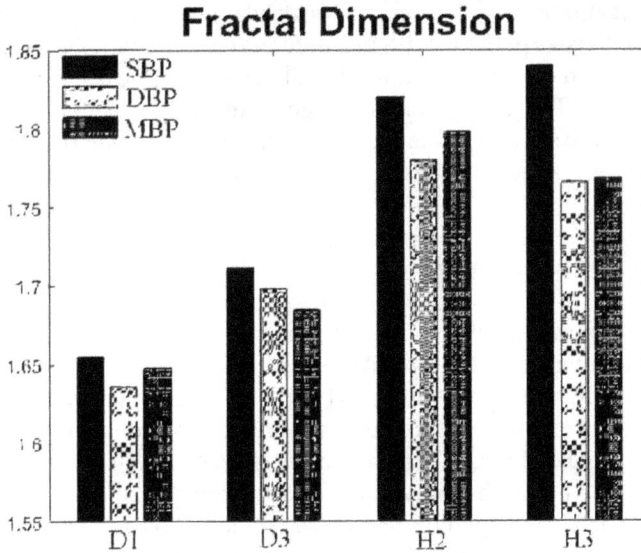

Figure 11.
Comparison of FD values of SBP, DBP, and MP in 4 hemodynamic classes [24]. *—p < 0.05.

FD value was determined for SBP, DBP, and mean BP (MBP, Hickam's formula) for patients of D1, D3, H2, and H3-classes; the duration of the daytime ABPM was 18–40 measurements, **Figure 11**.

Figure 11 shows significant differences (p < 0.05) in SBP signals of patients with the harmonic circulation phenotype (H2- and H3-classes) compared to patients with the dysfunctional diastolic circulation phenotype (D1- and D3-classes). Therefore, we considered FD for SBP signals as a potential marker of regulatory hemodynamic differences. **Figure 11** also shows a tendency for FD to increase in the hypertensive harmonic H3-class compared to the normotensive harmonic H2-class (norm), which is associated with a change in normal physiological reactions in the hypertensive harmonic H3-class caused by the action of the regulatory systems of cardiovascular control. In this case, the SBP signal exhibits more correlated or periodic behavior.

An opposite example is the loss of fractal dynamics (complexity of ABPM) and a decrease in FD values for the hypotensive dysfunctional diastolic D1-class, whose SBP time series are characterized by pronounced chaotic behavior due to a decrease (or complete absence) of cardiovascular control.

Analysis of clinical ABPM data showed that the FD value for SBP is limited from below by the threshold of FDd = 1.5 (random dynamics, minimal complexity of SBP, weakened or absent regulatory control of BP level, the cardiovascular system is poorly adapted to stress in everyday life). Low FD values are typical for pathological states of patients in D1-class, characteristic of patients in the intensive care unit with severe cardiovascular lesions and secondary hypotension.

The area of self-similar (fractal) dynamics of SBP is associated with the value of FDn ~ 1.8 (balance of cardiovascular regulation of BP level, maximum complexity of SBP signal). This FD value is associated with the hemodynamics of healthy patients in H2-class and a high degree of adaptability of the cardiovascular system. An increase in FD to the upper threshold value FDu = 2.0 (fully correlated SBP signal, strong cardiovascular regulation of BP level, but weak adaptation to stress in everyday life) is typical for hypertensive patients with harmonious circulation (H3-class).

It should be noted that the FD values for all hemodynamic classes exceed the lower threshold FDd = 1.5. Therefore, all ABPM signals are antipersistent (if a positive increase in SBP was recorded in the previous measurement, then there is a high probability of a negative increase in the current measurement and vice versa).

8. Discussion and conclusions

Our study was initiated by the main problems of AH treatment: the lack of reliable methods for detecting latent forms of AH and preclinical circulatory disorders; often insufficient or ineffective treatment of AH and achievement of the BP treatment target; low adherence of patients to the treatment of hypertension.

About 24-hour ABPM recordings (as well as HBPM over 24 hours) undoubtedly contain information about the individual characteristics of blood circulation, the accounting of which can help in solving these problems. We have developed a scientifically based analysis of blood circulation by linear regression modeling of ABPM data with the determination of the hemodynamic phenotype and class by regression coefficients, which makes it possible to differentiate the states of hypo- and hypertension, as well as potential applications in cardiology. To determine the phenotype, only 24-hour ABPM (or HBPM recording, 25–30 measurements over 7–10 days) is needed.

We studied the distribution of phenotypes in different categories of patients: healthy patients, patients with hypertension, coronary heart disease, stroke, and other diseases (more than 2500 patients of different ages). In hypertensive patients on antihypertensive pharmacotherapy, we analyzed the relationship of phenotypes with clinical and demographic factors and the probability of achieving the BP target, taking into account the pharmacotherapy used (number of drugs and pharmacological groups).

We have shown that hemodynamic phenotypes reflect patient blood circulation in the observed time interval (over a number of years). The change in phenotype is possible due to aging, diseases, lifestyle changes, etc., confirming that phenotype is a precise hemodynamic characteristic of the individual.

The main advantage of our method is that determining the hemodynamic phenotype is an important factor in prescribing the treatment of hypertension. For example, regardless of the pharmacological groups of drugs, patients with the D-phenotype are less likely to achieve the BP treatment target (31.2–45.2%) than patients with the H-phenotype (47.7–68.2%, $p < 0.05$). Additionally, patients with the D-phenotype have a lower QL, especially in the physical component ($p < 0.05$), and their QL decreases even more ($p < 0.05$) with the intensification of pharmacotherapy (≥ 2 drugs).

We found that the treatment of AH in patients with the D-phenotype should be comprehensive, using both psychotherapeutic and physiotherapeutic methods along with adjuvant drugs that improve vascular stiffness (vitamin D, statins, etc.) and psychoemotional status. In this case, pharmacotherapy requires drug combinations (especially fixed combinations), predominantly BB, ACE inhibitors, and thiazide/TLD. Patients with the D-phenotype should also be motivated to be physically active.

The proposed approach also reveals hidden circulatory disorders in normotensive people in the form of dysfunctional hemodynamic phenotypes and pathological classes of the harmonic phenotype: hypertensive class (H3) and transitional class to AH (H0).

These categories of patients need to be examined to exclude hidden forms of hypertension or other health disorders. We found that BB, CCB (especially in the absence of CIHD), and thiazide/TLD are most effective in pharmacotherapy for patients with the H-phenotype. For such patients, when using ACE inhibitors, the physical and mental components of QL should be corrected.

If normotensive healthy patients have dysfunctional phenotypes or "hypertensive" classes, their cardiovascular risk should be assessed by known factors (smoking, dyslipidemia, etc.), and recommendations should be made to change lifestyle and nutrition and to control BP and phenotype. If normotensive individuals have "hypertensive" classes of any phenotype, their cardiovascular risk should be assessed against known factors, and they should be screened for AH.

Furthermore, determining the hemodynamic phenotype in patients with OSA allows for predicting the effectiveness of CPAP therapy in terms of improving hemodynamic parameters and selecting patients for this specific and expensive method of treatment.

Determining the phenotype using the proposed method does not require special equipment and is available at any level of medical care, including outpatient therapeutic and general medical practice, cardiology, preventive medicine, sports and military medicine, functional diagnostics, and scientific research of blood circulation. It should be noted that patients have a very positive attitude toward the analysis of ABPM using our method, as it demonstrates an individual approach to the treatment of the patient.

Besides, it was the FD of the SBP that we considered as a parameter of the systemic autonomic regulation of BP levels. It should be noted that there is a tendency for FD to increase in the hypertensive harmonic H3-class compared to the normotensive harmonic H2-class, which is caused by hyper-regulation by the autonomic nervous system.

The opposite example is the loss of fractal dynamics (complexity of SBP) and a decrease in FD values for the hypotensive diastolic D1-class, which is characterized by pronounced chaotic behavior due to decreased (or absent, as in the case of ABPM of a heart transplant patient) cardiovascular control.

To assess the physiological state of the patient's blood circulation, we propose an integral indicator consisting of the nonlinear measure—the FD of SBP time series—and a qualitative variable—the individual hemodynamic class—determined by LRBPP on ABPM.

The data obtained indicate that further studies of hemodynamic phenotypes by the proposed method may be useful not only in hypertensive patients but also in different pathologies and different populations.

There are some limitations of this study: clinical studies of hemodynamic phenotypes and classes were conducted only on limited populations (in Belarus, Russia, and Poland). Also, we conducted studies that were limited in time, which does not allow us to draw conclusions about the prognostic significance of phenotypes over a long period of time (years, decades).

Our research is supported by patents of the Republic of Belarus (G 01 N 33/48: #4876; A 61B 5/02: #6950, #6952, #19833, #19976, #18998) and approved by the Belarus Ministry of Health (Method for determining the hemodynamic phenotype, No. 171-1218). In addition, the algorithm for hemodynamic classification developed by the authors is implemented in the software for ABPM apparatuses CARDIAN-MD and CARDIAN-SDM (Cardian, Belarus, https://cardian.by/). A special software unit diagnoses the phenotype of hemodynamics and visualizes individual regression coefficients on a diagnostic nomogram.

Author details

Margarita Voitikova[1*] and Raissa Khursa[2]

1 Institute of Physics, National Academy of Sciences of Belarus, Minsk, Belarus

2 Belarus State Medical University, Minsk, Belarus

*Address all correspondence to: m.voitikova@dragon.bas-net.by

IntechOpen

References

[1] Williams B, Mancia G, Spiering W, et al. 2018 ESC/ESH guidelines for the management of arterial hypertension. Journal of Hypertension. 2018;**36**(10): 1953-2041. DOI: 10.1097/HJH. 0000000000001940

[2] Rosenthal T. Prehypertension and the Cardiometabolic Syndrome. In: Zimlichman R, Julius S, Mancia G, editors. Prehypertension and the Cardiometabolic Syndrome. Cham: Springer; 2019. DOI: 10.1007/978-3-319-75310-2_5

[3] Cierpka-Kmiec K, Khursa R, Hering D. Hemodynamic phenotypes in chronic kidney disease patients based on linear regression of blood pressure parameters. Journal of Clinical Hypertension. 2024;**26**:1391-1401. DOI: 10.1111/jch.14880

[4] Karavaev AS, Ishbulatov YM, et al. Model of human cardiovascular system with a loop of autonomic regulation of the mean arterial pressure. Journal of the American Society of Hypertension. 2016;**10**(3):235-243. DOI: 10.1016/j. jash.2015.12.014

[5] Faini A, Parati G, Bilo G, Rienzo M. Di, Castiglioni P. Fractal characteristics of blood pressure and heart rate from ambulatory blood pressure monitored over 24-hours. In: Proceedings of the 2014 8th Conference of the European Study Group on Cardiovascular Oscillations (ESGCO), Trento, Italy. 25-28 May 2014. pp. 72-74. DOI: 10.1109/ ESGCO.2014.6847525

[6] Li Y, Wang JG, Dolan E, et al. Ambulatory arterial stiffness index derived from 24-hour ambulatory blood pressure monitoring. Hypertension. 2006;**47**:359-364. DOI: 10.1161/01. HYP.0000200695.34024.4c

[7] Dolan E, Thijs L, Li Y, Atkins N, McCormack P, McClory S, et al. Ambulatory arterial stiffness index as a predictor of cardiovascular mortality. Hypertension. 2006;**47**:365-370. DOI: 10.1161/01.HYP.0000200699.74641.c5

[8] Gavish B, Ben-Dov IZ, Bursztyn M. Linear relationship between systolic and diastolic blood pressure monitored over 24 h: Assessment and correlates. Journal of Hypertension. 2008;**26**:199-209

[9] Anokhin PK. Key Questions of a Theory of the Functional Systems. Moscow: Nauka; 1980

[10] Khursa RV. Hemodynamics phenotype by parameters of arterial pressure: Experience of clinical application. Zdravoohranenie. 2021;**5**: 37-51 (in Russian)

[11] Zaki MJ, Meira W Jr. Data Mining and Machine Learning: Fundamental Concepts and Algorithms (2nd ed.). Cambridge: Cambridge University Press; 2020

[12] Voitikova MV, Khursa RV. Classification of hemodynamics using a diagnostic Nomogram and ambulatory blood pressure data. Nonlinear Phenomena in Complex System. 2020;**13**(3):291-298. DOI: 10.33581/1561- 4085-2020-23-3-291-298

[13] Voitikova MV, Khursa RV. Analysis of 24-hour ambulatory blood pressure monitoring data using support vector machine. Nonlinear Phenomena in Complex Systems. 2014;**17**(1):50-56

[14] Voitikova MV, Khursa RV. Nomogram of hemodynamic states according to blood pressure parameters. Technologies of Living Systems. 2014;**2**:45-53 (in Russian)

[15] Voitikova MV, Khursa RV. Linear regression in haemodynamics. Nonlinear Phenomena in Complex Systems. 2012;**15**(2):203-206

[16] Voitikova MV, Voitovich AP, Khursa RV. The use of data mining for the classification of hemodynamic states. Physician and Information Technology. 2013;**1**:32-41 (in Russian)

[17] Moody GB, Mark RG. A database to support development and evaluation of intelligent intensive care monitoring. Computers in Cardiology. 1996;**23**:657-660 The MIMIC II Project database. Available from: https://physionet.org/content/mimic-ii/2.6.0/

[18] Khursa RV, Voitikova MV, Elinsky AA, Krupenin VP. Modern scientific advances in devices for 24-hour arterial pressure monitoring: New diagnostic capabilities. Medicine. 2018;**1**(100):25-30 (in Russian)

[19] Khursa R, Kezhun L. Hemodynamic phenotype and effects of vitamin D status correction in perimenopausal women with hypertension. Cardiology in Belarus. 2020;**12**(3):342-354

[20] Khursa RV, Voitikova MV, Stefański A, Wolf J, Narkiewicz K. Haemodynamic phenotypes and its association with blood pressure changes at continuous positive airway pressure therapy in obstructive sleep apnoea hypertensive patient. Arterial Hypertens. 2018;**22**(3):1-7. DOI: 10.5603/AH.a2018.0011

[21] Eke A, Herman P, Kocsis L, Kozak LR. Fractal characterization of complexity in temporal physiological signals. Physiological Measurement. 2002;**23**:R1-R38. DOI: 10.1088/0967-3334/23/1/201

[22] Armentano R, Legnani W, Cymerknop L. Fractal analysis of cardiovascular signals empowering the bioengineering knowledge. In: Fractal Analysis - Applications in Health Sciences and Social Sciences. London, UK: IntechOpen; 2017. DOI: 10.5772/67784

[23] Goldberger AL, Amaral LAN, Hausdorff JM, Ivanov PC, Peng C-K, Stanley HE. Fractal dynamics in physiology: Alterations with disease and aging. Proceedings of the National Academy of Sciences of the United States of America. 2002;**99**:2466-2472. DOI: 10.1073/pnas.012579499

[24] Voitikova M. Fractal Characterization and Modeling of Blood Pressure Signals. Proceedings of XXXI Annual International Seminar Nonlinear Phenomena in Complex Systems (NPCS). Nonlinear Dynamics and Applications. 2024;**30**:515-521

[25] Mandelbrot BB. The Fractal Geometry of Nature. New York: Freeman; 1982. 460 p

[26] Feder J. Fractals. New York: Plenum Press; 1988. 283 p

Chapter 4

Consequences of Hypertension

Abayomi Sanusi

Abstract

Through complex pathways that continue to be elucidated, hypertension damages tissues, organs and systems, and has become a public health risk factor and disease of global importance. Its mechanisms, complications on organ systems, and their salient features, are outlined to highlight how they could be understood to inform contemplating clinical, public health and policy strategies. Among these are: cardiac complications including coronary artery atherosclerosis, myocardial ischaemia and myocardial hypertrophy and its complications; cerebrovascular complications including haemorrhagic and ischaemic stroke; renal complications including and leading to end stage renal failure; vascular complications including aortic aneurysm and diffuse peripheral arterial disease; a wide range of ocular complications leading to and including complete and permanent vision loss. Ultimately, premature death can complicate untreated hypertension. More is needed to implement hypertension as the global public health issue it is and address its consequences.

Keywords: hypertension, complication, mechanisms, morbidity, mortality

1. Introduction

Blood pressure is the physical force generated by pulsatile myocardial contraction (systole) and relaxation (diastole) that compress blood against the internal walls of the arterial section of the circulatory system, and in combination with their compliance and flexibility propel blood to deliver a nearly steady flow at the level of the microvasculature to perfuse organs and tissues. It facilities the metabolic survival of cells, tissues and organs by enabling that the cellular level functions and interactions of electrolytes, minerals, nutrients and vital cells constituting blood plasma (which maintain the continuation of cellular vitality) are rarely sufficiently uninterrupted. Hence blood pressure drives the continuation of life.

Hypertension is persistently elevated blood pressure above thresholds optimal for the normal functioning of end organs, the continuation of which even without immediate complications will trigger a cascade of long-term complications. A widely utilised clinic based diagnostic threshold for metabolically healthy human adults is systolic pressure of 140 mmHg (millimetres of mercury) and diastolic pressure of 90 mmHg [1]. **Table 1** outlines the diagnostic definition and classification of hypertension based on guidelines used in Europe, North America, and much of the rest of the world [2, 3]. Diagnostic threshold and management decisions in clinical practice, although technically informed by local, national and international guidelines, are often based on individual patient characteristics and circumstances including age and existing medical conditions [2, 4, 5].

IntechOpen

ACCA/AHA[a] 2017

Category	SBP[c] (mmHg)		DBP[d] (mmHg)
Normal	<120	&	<80
Elevated	120–129	&	<80
Stage 1 hypertension	130–139	/	80–89
Stage 2 hypertension	≥140	/	≥90

ESC/ESH[b] 2023

Category	SBP[c] (mmHg)		DBP[d] (mmHg)
Optimal	<120	&	<80
Normal	120–129	&/	80–84
High normal	130–139	&/	85–89
Grade 1 hypertension	140–159	&/	90–99
Grade 2 hypertension	160–179	&/	100–109
Grade 3 hypertension	≥180	&/	≥110
Isolated systolic hypertension	≥140	&	<90
Isolated diastolic hypertension	<140	&	≥90

Level of BP[e] defining hypertension by measurement type

ACCA/AHA 2017

Measurement type	SBP (mmHg)		DBP (mmHg)
Office/clinic BP[f] (attended)	≥130	&	≥80
Home BP[e] mean	≥130	&	≥80
Daytime mean, ABPM[g]	≥130	&/	≥80
24 hour mean, ABPM[g]	≥125		≥75
Night time mean, ABPM[g]	≥110		≥65

ESC/ESH 2023

Measurement type	SBP (mmHg)		DBP (mmHg)
Office/clinic BP (attended)	≥140	&/	≥90
Home BP mean	≥135		≥85
Daytime mean, ABPM	≥135		≥85
24 hour mean, ABPM	≥130		≥80
Night time mean, ABPM	≥120		≥70

[a] ACCA/AHA: *American College of Cardiology/American Heart Association.*
[b] ESC/ESH: *European Society of Cardiology/European Society of Hypertension.*
[c] SBP: *Systolic Blood Pressure.*
[d] DBP: *Diastolic Blood Pressure.*
[e] BP: *Blood Pressure.*
[f] Office/clinic BP: *attended by healthcare professional.*
[g] ABPM: *Ambulatory Blood Pressure Monitor.*

Table 1.
Definition and classification of hypertension.

Less than a century ago hypertension was more prevalent in Western countries with the most industrialised economies, but has become increasingly more prevalent in less industrialised countries and in every region of the world [6–8]. Today with more than 1.1 billion people hypertensive globally, hypertension has become an important global public health challenge [9, 10]. However, given the remarkable compensatory capacity of the cardiovascular and neuroendocrine systems, hypertension displays a quiescent, painless, relatively asymptomatic course over long durations that may stretch from multiple years to decades. It therefore has the potential to be both "accidentally" and "conveniently" ignored compared to inflammatory or painful conditions receiving immediate attention, and neoplastic conditions demanding urgency. This disfavourable pattern of attention toward "the silent killer" is in keeping with the projection that hypertension will continue to be responsible for the highest global mortality rates beyond 2030 [10, 11].

Hence globally, only a minority of people with hypertension is aware that they have it. Only a minority of people with awareness of their hypertension actively treats it. And only a minority of people undergoing hypertension treatment achieve hypertension control [12, 13]. By implication only a minority of global hypertension cases are controlled, meaning that the vast majority of people with hypertension live with uncontrolled hypertension. So, globally, most hypertensive individuals, irrespective of their awareness of hypertension, or their capability or opportunity to monitor or manage it, live with uncontrolled hypertension.

In considering the consequences of hypertension it is important to understand relevant individual risk factors. Among the risk factors are old age, ethnicity, overweight or obesity, a sedentary lifestyle or one lacking in sufficient physical activity, smoking, excessive dietary salt, alcohol consumption, and metabolic disease such as diabetes mellitus [14, 15].

Understanding the implications of uncontrolled hypertension is relevant to quality of life, morbidity and premature deaths. It is important to inform, guide or customise clinical management, and also to shape and influence public health strategies and policy. In this chapter, the main physiological consequences of uncontrolled hypertension due to unrecognised, unmanaged or poorly managed hypertension are presented.

2. Mechanisms of the complications

Multiple factors including genetics, advancing age, lifestyle and existing systemic disease contribute to hypertension and trigger a combination of sympathetic hyperactivity and neurohormonal dysregulation, including increased renin-angiotensin-aldosterone axis activation [16, 17]. Over time these cause structural alterations, notably, irreversible large artery stiffening. Multiple mechanisms mediate this. Dysfunction of the innermost layer, the intima, is mediated by reduced endothelial nitric oxide production, alterations in the vascular smooth muscle cell cytoskeleton, and calcifications associated with atherosclerosis [18].

Several dysfunctions contribute to arterial stiffening attributed to the middle layer, the media. Among these are irreparable elastin degradation caused by cyclic mechanical fatigue over time, elastase-mediated proteolysis, intimal calcification and inflammation [19]. Dysfunction of the outermost adventitial layer contributes to arterial stiffening through collagen deposition and calcification [19, 20]. The resulting irreversible arterial stiffening manifest as increased arterial pressure and excess pulsatility, which over time causes repetitive microvascular trauma to the richly per-fused low-resistance vascular beds of end organs, and eventual organ failure [19, 21].

All organ tissues directly or indirectly rely on normal blood pressure for optimal physiology, and experience a degree of dysfunction when hypertension is sustained for sufficiently prolonged durations. Recognition and quantification of resulting dysfunctions rely on the capability of the individual physiological reserves of tissue-organs, and the acuteness or tolerability of the associated symptoms or detectable signs.

In addition to being the main cause of death from cardiovascular disease through myocardial infarction, cerebrovascular ischaemia and haemorrhage [22], hyperten-sion is also a well-established independent risk for deaths from chronic renal failure and heart failure [23–25], and is associated with the dysfunction of several organ systems.

3. Cardiac complications

Coronary artery atherosclerosis directly complicates hypertension with the consequence of myocardial ischaemia, which subsequently progresses to infarction. Atherosclerosis is the accumulation of aggregates of lesions consisting of lipids, cho-lesterol, inflammatory cells and calcium as plaques within arterial walls. These nar-row arterial lumen, contributing to myocardial ischaemia. Atherosclerosis is systemic, and macroscopic atheromatous plaques can start as early in life as infancy [26, 27], but may take decades to progress and become symptomatic [28]. Hypertension is known to accelerate coronary atherosclerosis through its pro-inflammatory effects on small and large arteries [29, 30]; but multiple molecular and cellular level mecha-nisms continue to be unravelled [31]. Atherosclerotic plaques are reversible [32] but can also progress rapidly [28, 33].

Hypertension creates additional haemodynamic stress, which the myocardium has to compensate. Over time, the myocardium hypertrophies, progresses to varying degrees of myocardial dysfunction, severe disability and ultimately death [14, 34]. The end stage of most heart disease is heart failure, for which hypertension is both a cause and risk factor [35]. Its epidemiology is evolving with its prevalence increas-ing among young people in association with increasing obesity, and in low to middle income countries in association with increasing adoption of Western lifestyles that increase the risk of hypertension [36]. Heart failure remains a debilitating, steady and efficient killer whose molecular mechanisms remain to be fully understood [37].

4. Cerebrovascular complications

Alongside cardiovascular consequences, the most commonly recognised complica-tion of hypertension is stroke, or cerebrovascular ischaemia from occlusive atheroma-tous plaques, thrombi or a haemorrhage. Depending on severity and distribution of the involved vessels, cerebrovascular ischaemia can be immediately fatal, or with interven-tion partly resolve but with varying severities of often devastating or challenging cog-nitive, autonomic nervous, sensorineural and musculoskeletal sequelae [38]. Untreated hypertension increases this risk by accelerating carotid atherosclerosis [25, 39].

Cerebrovascular atherosclerosis may initially present as Transient Ischemic Attacks, with partial incomplete and reversible symptoms of central nervous system ischaemia. Longer-term complications include Vascular Dementia, and more significant cognitive impairment [40–43].

It remains a leading cause of death and neurological disability in countries of all income levels, although low- and middle-income countries bear the heaviest burden. Similarly, in high-income countries, huge disparities remain along racial, ethnic and socioeconomic demarcations [44, 45].

5. Renal complications

Hypertension is both a cause and complication of chronic kidney disease. It contributes to chronic kidney disease while chronic kidney disease complicates hypertension through dysfunction in the regulation of sympathetic activity, inflammation and sodium excretion [46, 47].

The consequences of chronic kidney failure resulting from hypertension are indistinguishable from causes from other aetiologies. It is a progressive failure in the efficiency of glomerular function. A practical definition widely used in clinical practice is the presence of either or both of a glomerular filtration rate of less than 60 mL/min per 1.73 m^2, and clinical or biochemical markers of kidney damage for at least 3 months duration [48].

Accumulation of metabolites results in a complex cluster of complications associated with significant reduction in quality of life, and almost invariably ends up in premature death or end-stage renal disease. Common complications include disturbances in metabolism of vitamin D, calcium and phosphate; and anaemia due to impaired erythropoietin production, impaired red blood cell survival and iron deficiency. Ultimately chronic kidney failure is progressive, irreversible and incurable [48, 49]. Globally the prevalence of chronic kidney failure progression to end stage kidney disease is rising [50–52].

6. Vascular complications

Aside accelerating atherosclerosis thereby contributing to and complicating cerebrovascular, coronary arterial and renal disease, hypertension is also a major risk factor for aortic aneurysm and diffuse peripheral arterial disease [25, 53]. Mortality from aortic aneurysm is on the increase, although best explained by increasing age [54]. Peripheral arterial disease, typified by atherosclerotic occlusive disease of the arterial supply to the lower limbs, is an important cause of ischaemic limb loss, and contributes to reduced quality of life and premature deaths [55–58]. It is increasingly prevalent with advancing age, constituting an important disease burden [59, 60], following the pattern of epidemiological transition to chronic, metabolic and atherogenic diseases [61, 62].

Perhaps one of the most notable characteristics of peripheral arterial disease is that by the time peripheral arterial disease becomes clinically symptomatic, other manifestations of uncontrolled or inadequately controlled hypertension and the contributing risk factors are likely to already be symptomatic too. Hence the possibility of any treatment, especially invasive treatments, may be determined by the existing physiological capability to tolerate them. This means that established comorbidities, especially where multiple and severe, are influential in determining the feasibility, tolerability or logic of treating peripheral arterial disease at all. Where treatment is precluded or unadvisable due to physiological frailty, alternative choice may be made of best palliation and symptomatic support with understanding of progression to limb loss and premature death.

7. Ocular complications

Hypertension is responsible for a wide range of often subtle retinal vascular degenerative changes collectively termed hypertensive retinopathy which ultimately lead to partial or complete blindness [63–65]. These include hypertensive choroidopathy-variable patterns of retinal arteriolar stenoses and arteriovenous crossing changes compromising retinal vascular bed autoregulation, leading to ischaemia, necrosis and retinal detachment [66]. Others include retinal venous occlusion retinal arteriolar embolism, macroaneurysm, haemorrhage, optic neuropathy, and optic disc and macular oedema [67, 68].

Hypertension is understood to not be directly responsible for, but contributory to diabetic retinopathy, glaucoma, and age-related macular degeneration. The associations are not fully elucidated but may partly be via common risk factors, and their management and age [69, 70].

The most important factor underlying the range of hypertension-induced conditions that lead to blindness may be the irreplaceability of the retina. While hypertension itself is preventable and mostly reversible, the direct vascular causes of retinal ischaemia, most notably central arterial occlusion, is rarely treatable [71], retinal degeneration remains incurable [72] and the underlying mechanisms of indirect retinal ischaemia remain inadequately understood [73]. The implications of visual loss for quality of life cannot be underestimated despite ocular hypertension complications being not emergently or directly fatal like cerebrovascular and cardiac emergencies.

8. Mitigating the complications

World Health Organisation recommendations to address hypertension include: integrating hypertension prevention and other chronic disease reduction strategies at the primary care level; funding such integrated chronic disease strategies; providing basic diagnostic tools and medication; reducing risk factors in the population; workplace based wellness programmes; and monitoring [10]. These, and similar recommendations demand large amounts of resources. Risk factor mitigation programmes such as awareness, education, lifestyle, diet, physical activity and stress management interventions demand significant resources and organisation. Notwithstanding the depths of resources available to healthcare and public health systems, effective early detection and diagnosis through screening programmes potentially demand challenging levels of organisation and resources. Similarly, promptly initiated, evidence based, cost-efficient and appropriately followed up pharmacological intervention remains elusive for most populations in most of the world. Hence, globally, effective and efficient prevention of the complications of hypertension remain elusive.

9. Looking forward

The World Health Organisation recommendations for addressing hypertension are comprehensive, but globally a lot of work remains to be done to address primary hypertension prevention through risk factor reduction. This applies to countries less capable of addressing hypertension because of inadequate healthcare infrastructure and resources; and those better able to provide pharmacological treatments alike. Among the consequences are that the true severity and impact of the global hypertension endemic does not appear matched by efforts. As such, there are no known examples of healthcare or public health systems that have completely democratised early hypertension detection and management such that its populations achieve equally good hypertension outcomes irrespective of socioeconomic status.

10. Conclusion

Hypertension is both an independent systemic disease and a potent risk factor for cardiovascular and cerebrovascular diseases. Its renal, peripheral vascular and ocular complications comprise a wide range of conditions with underlying limitation of effective tissue perfusion that impair normal physiology thereby imposing disabilities, limit quality of life and contribute to premature death.

Cardiac complications vary from nonspecific symptoms related to invisible atherosclerotic coronary artery disease to myocardial ischaemia to heart failure and consequent psychological and physical disability to death.

Cerebrovascular complications include Transient Ischaemic Attack, stroke, varying severities of autonomic nervous, sensorineural and musculoskeletal disabilities. Renal complications lead to end stage renal failure. Peripheral vascular complications lead to limb loss. Ocular complications ultimately lead to blindness. Given the systemic nature of hypertension, multiple complications may develop concurrently, interact to exacerbate each other and contribute to adverse psychological health and poorer quality of life.

Hypertension's consequences, including the adverse quality of life and psychological impacts of stroke, cardiac and renal failure, can be challenging to quantify, [74–78].

It is clear that the disruption of normal physiology, exhaustive description of resulting pathological processes, the disease entities and complex symptoms constituting the complications of hypertension through which it limit tissue, organ and system physiology cannot be exhaustively covered in this text.

This text has presented how they impair quality of life, cause premature deaths, and given an insight into how extensive they can be as individual pathologies that they cannot be exhaustively covered in this text (Refer to the relevant chapters of the book).

Given that unknown, yet to be understood and misattributed complications also cannot be quantified nor contribute to our current understanding of the consequences of hypertension, the true cost of hypertension may be difficult to accurately estimate. Perhaps the critical challenge is that despite hypertension being understood as predictable, preventable, manageable and often treatable, and its risk factors well known; it remains, through and in combination with cardiovascular diseases, responsible for the highest number of deaths for multiple decades.

Conflict of interest

The author declares no conflict of interest.

Author details

Abayomi Sanusi
Department of Health Sciences, The University of York, United Kingdom

*Address all correspondence to: abayomi.sanusi@york.ac.uk

IntechOpen

References

[1] Volpe M, Gallo G, Modena MG, Ferri C, Desideri G, Tocci G. Updated recommendations on cardiovascular prevention in 2022: An executive document of the Italian Society of Cardiovascular Prevention. High Blood Pressure & Cardiovascular Prevention. 2022;**2022**:1-12

[2] Brunström M, Burnier M, Grassi G, Januszewicz A, Muiesan M, Tsioufis K, et al. ESH Guidelines for the management of arterial hypertension The Task Force for the management of arterial hypertension of the European Society of Hypertension. Endorsed by the International Society of Hypertension (ISH) and the European Renal Association (ERA). Journal of Hypertension. 2023;**41**:13-24

[3] Liew CH, McEvoy JW. Cardiovascular risk prevention in clinical medicine: Current guidelines in the United States and in Europe. In: Chirinos JA, editor. Textbook of Arterial Stiffness and Pulsatile Hemodynamics in Health and Disease. London, United Kingdom: Academic Press; 2022

[4] Chobanian AV, Bakris GL, Black HR, Cushman WC, Green LA, Izzo JL, et al. Seventh report of the joint National Committee on prevention, detection, evaluation, and treatment of high blood pressure. Hypertension. 2003;**42**:1206-1252. DOI: 10.1161/01. HYP.0000107251.49515.c2

[5] Unger T, Borghi C, Charchar F, Khan NA, Poulter NR, Prabhakaran D, et al. 2020 International Society of Hypertension Global Hypertension Practice Guidelines. Hypertension. 2020;**75**:1334-1357. DOI: 10.1161/ HYPERTENSIONAHA.120.15026

[6] Donnison CP. Blood pressure in the African native. Its bearing upon the aetiology of hyperpiesia and arterio-sclerosis. Lancet. 1929:6-7

[7] Abrahams D, Alele C. A clinical study of hypertensive disease in West Africa. West African Medical of Journal. 1960;**9**:183-193

[8] Vint FW. Post-mortem findings in the natives of Kenya. East African Medical Journal. 1937;**13**:332-344

[9] Li Y, Cao G, Jing W, Liu J, Liu M. Global trends and regional differences in incidence and mortality of cardiovascular disease, 1990– 2019: Findings from 2019 global burden of disease study. European Journal of Preventive Cardiology. 2023;**30**:276-286

[10] World Health Organization. A Global Brief on Hypertension: Silent Killer, Global Public Health Crisis: World Health Day 2013. Geneva: World Health Organization; 2013

[11] World Health Organization. Global Report on Hypertension: The Race against a Silent Killer. Geneva: World Health Organization; 2023

[12] GBD 2015 Risk Factors Collaborators. Global, regional, and national comparative risk assessment of 79 behavioural, environmental and occupational, and metabolic risks or clusters of risks, 1990-2015: A systematic analysis for the Global Burden of Disease Study 2015. The Lancet (London, England). 2016;**388**:1659

[13] Chow CK, Teo KK, Rangarajan S, Islam S, Gupta R, Avezum A, et al. Prevalence, awareness, treatment, and control of hypertension in rural and

urban communities in high-, middle-, and low-income countries. Journal of the American Medical Association. 2013;**310**:959-968

[14] Masenga SK, Kirabo A. Hypertensive heart disease: Risk factors, complications and mechanisms. Frontiers in Cardiovascular Medicine. 2023;**10**:1205475. DOI: 10.3389/fcvm.2023.1205475

[15] Roumie CL, Hung AM, Russell GB, Basile J, Kreider KE, Nord J, et al. Blood pressure control and the association with diabetes mellitus incidence: Results from SPRINT randomized trial. Hypertension. 2020;**75**:331-338. DOI: 10.1161/HYPERTENSIONAHA.118.12572

[16] Takahashi H, Yoshika M, Komiyama Y, Nishimura M. The central mechanism underlying hypertension: A review of the roles of sodium ions, epithelial sodium channels, the renin–angiotensin–aldosterone system, oxidative stress and endogenous digitalis in the brain. Hypertension Research. 2011;**34**:1147-1160

[17] Hall JE. Control of blood pressure by the renin-angiotensin-aldosterone system. Clinical Cardiology. 1991;**14**:6-21. DOI: 10.1002/clc.4960141802

[18] Duca L, Blaise S, Romier B, Laffargue M, Gayral S, El Btaouri H, et al. Matrix ageing and vascular impacts: Focus on elastin fragmentation. Cardiovascular Research. 2016;**110**:298-308. DOI: 10.1093/cvr/cvw061

[19] Chirinos JA, Segers P, Hughes T, Townsend R. Large-artery stiffness in health and disease: JACC state-of-the-art review. Journal of the American College of Cardiology. 2019;**74**:1237-1263

[20] Araújo, Passos LS, Becker-Greene D, Aikawa E. Mechanisms of calcification in the aortic wall and aortic valve. In: Textbook of Arterial Stiffness and Pulsatile Hemodynamics in Health and Disease. Cambridge, MA, USA: Academic Press; 2022. pp. 327-340. DOI: 10.1016/B978-0-323-91391-1.00021-2

[21] Chirinos JA, editor. Hemodynamic role of the aorta. In: Textbook of Arterial Stiffness and Pulsatile Hemodynamics in Health and Disease. Cambridge, MA, USA: Academic Press; 2022. pp. 155-168. DOI: 10.1016/B978-0-323-91391-1.00010-8

[22] Arima H, Barzi F, Chalmers J. Mortality patterns in hypertension. Journal of Hypertension. 2011;**29**:S3-S7. DOI: 10.1097/01.hjh.0000410246.59221.b1

[23] Verdecchia P, Angeli F, Gattobigio R, Rapicetta C, Reboldi G. Impact of blood pressure variability on cardiac and cerebrovascular complications in hypertension. American Journal of Hypertension. 2007;**20**:154-161

[24] Levy D, Garrison RJ, Savage DD, Kannel WB, Castelli WP. Prognostic implications of echocardiographically determined left ventricular mass in the Framingham Heart Study. New England Journal of Medicine. 1990;**322**:1561-1566

[25] Doyle AE. Hypertension and vascular disease. American Journal of Hypertension. 1991;**4**:103S-106S

[26] Takei H, Strong JP, Yutani C, Malcom GT. Comparison of coronary and aortic atherosclerosis in youth from Japan and the USA. Atherosclerosis. 2005;**180**:171-179. DOI: 10.1016/j.atherosclerosis.2004.11.014

[27] Imakita M, Yutani C, Strong JP, Sakurai I, Sumiyoshi A, Watanabe T, et al. Second nation-wide study of atherosclerosis in infants, children and young adults in Japan. Atherosclerosis.

2001;**155**:487-497. DOI: 10.1016/
S0021-9150(00)00595-5

[28] Fan J, Watanabe T. Atherosclerosis: Known and unknown. Pathology International. 2022;**72**:151-160. DOI: 10.1111/pin.13202

[29] Hollander W. Role of hypertension in atherosclerosis and cardiovascular disease. The American Journal of Cardiology. 1976;**38**:786-800. DOI: 10.1016/0002-9149(76)90357-X

[30] Chobanian AV. Exacerbation of atherosclerosis by hypertension: Potential mechanisms and clinical implications. Archives of Internal Medicine. 1996;**156**:1952. DOI: 10.1001/archinte.1996.00440160064009

[31] Frąk W, Wojtasińska A, Lisińska W, Młynarska E, Franczyk B, Rysz J. Pathophysiology of cardiovascular diseases: New insights into molecular mechanisms of atherosclerosis, arterial hypertension, and coronary artery disease. Biomedicine. 2022;**10**:1938. DOI: 10.3390/biomedicines10081938

[32] Parsons C, Agasthi P, Mookadam F, Arsanjani R. Reversal of coronary atherosclerosis: Role of life style and medical management. Trends in Cardiovascular Medicine. 2018;**28**:524-531. DOI: 10.1016/j.tcm.2018.05.002

[33] Neglia D, Caselli C, Maffei E, Cademartiri F, Meloni A, Bossone E, et al. Rapid plaque progression is independently associated with hyperglycemia and low HDL cholesterol in patients with stable coronary artery disease: A PARADIGM study. Circulation: Cardiovascular Imaging. 2024;**17**(7):e016481. DOI: 10.1161/CIRCIMAGING.123.016481

[34] Messerli FH, Rimoldi SF, Bangalore S. The transition from hypertension to heart failure. JACC: Heart Failure. 2017;**5**:543-551. DOI: 10.1016/j.jchf.2017.04.012

[35] Roger VL. Epidemiology of heart failure: A contemporary perspective. Circulation Research. 2021;**128**:1421-1434. DOI: 10.1161/CIRCRESAHA.121.318172

[36] Groenewegen A, Rutten FH, Mosterd A, Hoes AW. Epidemiology of heart failure. European Journal of Heart Failure. 2020;**22**:1342-1356. DOI: 10.1002/ejhf.1858

[37] Lippi G, Sanchis-Gomar F. Global epidemiology and future trends of heart failure. AME Medical Journal. 2020;**5**:15-15. DOI: 10.21037/amj.2020.03.03

[38] Storey CE, Pols H. A history of cerebrovascular disease. In: Handbook of Clinical Neurology. Toronto: Elsevier; 2009. pp. 401-415. DOI: 10.1016/S0072-9752(08)02127-1

[39] Cuspidi C, Sala C, Tadic M, Rescaldani M, De Giorgi GA, Grassi G, et al. Untreated masked hypertension and carotid atherosclerosis: A meta-analysis. Blood Pressure. 2015;**24**:65-71. DOI: 10.3109/00365521.2014.992185

[40] Bir SC, Khan MW, Javalkar V, Toledo EG, Kelley RE. Emerging concepts in vascular dementia: A review. Journal of Stroke and Cerebrovascular Diseases. 2021;**30**:105864. DOI: 10.1016/j.jstrokecerebrovasdis.2021.105864

[41] Sachdev PS, Brodaty H, Valenzuela MJ, Lorentz L, Looi JCL, Berman K, et al. Clinical determinants of dementia and mild cognitive impairment following ischaemic stroke: The Sydney stroke study. Dementia and Geriatric Cognitive Disorders. 2006;**21**:275-283. DOI: 10.1159/000091434

[42] Ivan CS, Seshadri S, Beiser A, Au R, Kase CS, Kelly-Hayes M, et al. Dementia after stroke: The Framingham study. Stroke. 2004;**35**:1264-1268. DOI: 10.1161/01. STR.0000127810.92616.78

[43] Rost NS, Meschia JF, Gottesman R, Wruck L, Helmer K, Greenberg SM, et al. Cognitive impairment and dementia after stroke: Design and rationale for the DISCOVERY study. Stroke. 2021;**52**:e499-e516

[44] Prust ML, Forman R, Ovbiagele B. Addressing disparities in the global epidemiology of stroke. Nature Reviews Neurology. 2024;**20**:207-221

[45] Feigin VL, Nichols E, Alam T, Bannick MS, Beghi E, Blake N, et al. Global, regional, and national burden of neurological disorders, 1990-2016: A systematic analysis for the Global Burden of Disease Study 2016. The Lancet Neurology. 2019;**18**:459-480. DOI: 10.1016/S1474-4422(18)30499-X

[46] Hamrahian SM, Falkner B. Hypertension in chronic kidney disease. Hypertension: From Basic Research to Clinical Practice. Cham: Springer; 2017:307-325. DOI: 10.1007/5584_2017_30

[47] Huan Y, Cohen DL, Townsend RR. Pathophysiology of hypertension in chronic kidney disease. In: Chronic Renal Disease. Philadelphia, PA, USA: Elsevier; 2015. pp. 163-169. DOI: 10.1016/ B978-0-12-411602-3.00014-7

[48] Webster AC, Nagler EV, Morton RL, Masson P. Chronic kidney disease. The Lancet. 2017;**389**:1238-1252. DOI: 10.1016/S0140-6736(16)32064-5

[49] Kalantar-Zadeh K, Jafar TH, Nitsch D, Neuen BL, Perkovic V. Chronic kidney disease. The Lancet.

2021;**398**:786-802. DOI: 10.1016/ S0140-6736(21)00519-5

[50] El Nahas AM, Bello AK. Chronic kidney disease: The global challenge. The Lancet. 2005;**365**:331-340. DOI: 10.1016/S0140-6736(05)17789-7

[51] Udani S, Lazich I, Bakris GL. Epidemiology of hypertensive kidney disease. Nature Reviews. Nephrology. 2011;**7**:11-21. DOI: 10.1038/ nrneph.2010.154

[52] Collins AJ, Foley RN, Chavers B, Gilbertson D, Herzog C, Johansen K, et al. US Renal Data System 2011 Annual Data Report. American Journal of Kidney Diseases. 2012;**59**:A7. DOI: 10.1053/j. ajkd.2011.11.015

[53] Chobanian AV. Vascular effects of systemic hypertension. The American Journal of Cardiology. 1992;**69**:3-7. DOI: 10.1016/0002-9149(92)90010-V

[54] Krafcik BM, Stone DH, Cai M, Jarmel IA, Eid M, Goodney PP, et al. Changes in global mortality from aortic aneurysm. Journal of Vascular Surgery. 2024;**80**:81-88.e1. DOI: 10.1016/j. jvs.2024.02.025

[55] Anand SS, Caron F, Eikelboom JW, Bosch J, Dyal L, Aboyans V, et al. Major adverse limb events and mortality in patients with peripheral artery disease: The COMPASS trial. Journal of the American College of Cardiology. 2018;**71**:2306-2315

[56] Clement D, De Buyzere M, Duprez D. Hypertension in peripheral arterial disease. Current Pharmaceutical Design. 2004;**10**:3615-3620. DOI: 10.2174/1381612043382819

[57] Hess CN, Huang Z, Patel MR, Baumgartner I, Berger JS, Blomster JI, et al. Acute limb ischemia in

peripheral artery disease: Insights from EUCLID. Circulation. 2019;**140**:556-565. DOI: 10.1161/ CIRCULATIONAHA.119.039773

[58] Golomb BA, Dang TT, Criqui MH. Peripheral arterial disease: Morbidity and mortality implications. Circulation. 2006;**114**:688-699. DOI: 10.1161/ CIRCULATIONAHA.105.593442

[59] Selvin E, Erlinger TP. Prevalence of and risk factors for peripheral arterial disease in the United States: Results from the National Health and Nutrition Examination Survey, 1999-2000. Circulation. 2004;**110**:738-743

[60] Norgren L, Hiatt WR, Dormandy JA, Nehler MR, Harris KA, Fowkes FGR, et al. Inter-society consensus for the management of peripheral arterial disease (TASC II). Journal of Vascular Surgery. 2007;**45**:S5-S67

[61] Horváth L, Németh N, Fehér G, Kívés Z, Endrei D, Boncz I. Epidemiology of peripheral artery disease: Narrative review. Life. 2022;**12**:1041. DOI: 10.3390/ life12071041

[62] Fowkes FGR, Aboyans V, Fowkes FJ, McDermott MM, Sampson UK, Criqui MH. Peripheral artery disease: Epidemiology and global perspectives. Nature Reviews Cardiology. 2017;**14**:156-170

[63] Wong TY, Mitchell P. Hypertensive retinopathy. New England Journal of Medicine. 2004;**351**:2310-2317

[64] Konstantinidis L, Guex-Crosier Y. Hypertension and the eye. Current Opinion in Ophthalmology. 2016;**27**:514-521

[65] Bhargava M, Ikram M, Wong TY. How does hypertension affect your eyes? Journal of Human Hypertension. 2012;**26**:71-83

[66] Wolffsohn JS, Hurcomb PG. Hypertension and the eye. Current Hypertension Reports. 2002;**4**:471-476

[67] Katsi V, Marketou M, Vlachopoulos C, Tousoulis D, Souretis G, Papageorgiou N, et al. Impact of arterial hypertension on the eye. Current Hypertension Reports. 2012;**14**:581-590. DOI: 10.1007/s11906-012-0283-6

[68] Central Vein Occlusion Study Group. Natural history and clinical management of central retinal vein occlusion. Archives of Ophthalmology. 1997;**115**:486-491

[69] Drance SM. Some factors in the production of low tension glaucoma. The British Journal of Ophthalmology. 1972;**56**:229

[70] Group UPDS. Tight blood pressure control and risk of macrovascular and microvascular complications in type 2 diabetes: UKPDS 38. BMJ. British Medical Journal. 1998;**317**:703-713

[71] Daruich A, Robert MP, Zola M, Matet A, Bremond-Gignac D. Retinal stroke: Research models, targets and experimental drugs. Expert Opinion on Investigational Drugs. 2023;**32**:755-760. DOI: 10.1080/13543784.2023.2254688

[72] Yang S, Zhou J, Li D. Functions and diseases of the retinal pigment epithelium. Frontiers in Pharmacology. 2021;**12**:727870. DOI: 10.3389/ fphar.2021.727870

[73] Mohite AA, Perais JA, McCullough P, Lois N. Retinal ischaemia in diabetic retinopathy: Understanding and overcoming a therapeutic challenge. Journal of Clinical Medicine. 2023;**12**:2406. DOI: 10.3390/ jcm12062406

[74] Khedr EM, Abdelrahman AA, Desoky T, Zaki AF, Gamea A. Post-stroke

depression: Frequency, risk factors, and impact on quality of life among 103 stroke patients—Hospital-based study. The Egyptian Journal of Neurology Psychiatry Neurosurgery. 2020;**56**:66. DOI: 10.1186/s41983-020-00199-8

[75] Xu X, Rao Y, Shi Z, Liu L, Chen C, Zhao Y. Hypertension impact on health-related quality of life: A cross-sectional survey among middle-aged adults in Chongqing, China. International Journal of Hypertension. 2016;**2016**:7404957

[76] Bailey PK, Hamilton AJ, Clissold RL, Inward CD, Caskey FJ, Ben-Shlomo Y, et al. Young adults' perspectives on living with kidney failure: A systematic review and thematic synthesis of qualitative studies. BMJ Open. 2018;**8**:e019926. DOI: 10.1136/bmjopen-2017-019926

[77] Minshall C, Ski CF, Apputhurai P, Thompson DR, Castle DJ, Jenkins Z, et al. Exploring the impact of illness perceptions, self-efficacy, coping strategies, and psychological distress on quality of life in a post-stroke cohort. Journal of Clinical Psychology in Medical Settings. 2021;**28**:174-180. DOI: 10.1007/s10880-020-09700-0

[78] Zambrano J, Celano CM, Januzzi JL, Massey CN, Chung W, Millstein RA, et al. Psychiatric and psychological interventions for depression in patients with heart disease: A scoping review. Journal of the American Heart Association. 2020;**9**:e018686. DOI: 10.1161/JAHA.120.018686

Chapter 5

Secondary Hypertension

Titus F. Msoka

Abstract

The secondary hypertension chapter provides a comprehensive overview of secondary hypertension, a significant form of high blood pressure that arises due to identifiable underlying conditions, distinguishing it from primary hypertension, which has no known cause. Secondary hypertension is more frequently observed in younger populations and often presents as treatment-resistant, necessitating careful evaluation for effective management. The chapter categorizes various causes, including renal disorders, endocrine abnormalities such as primary aldosteronism and Cushing's syndrome, and other contributors, like sleep-disordered breathing, coarctation of the aorta, and certain medications. The critical importance of accurate diagnosis is emphasized, highlighting the role of advanced imaging and biochemical tests in uncovering these underlying conditions. Treatment approaches are discussed, including lifestyle changes, targeted pharmacotherapy tailored to the specific etiology, and the consideration of surgical interventions for certain conditions, such as renal artery stenosis or adrenal tumors. Prognostic outcomes vary based on the reversibility of the underlying condition and the effectiveness of treatment strategies. For instance, conditions like pheochromocytoma may lead to significant remission of hypertension post-treatment, whereas chronic conditions require long-term management. The chapter ultimately underscores the importance of early detection of the cause of secondary hypertension, patient adherence to treatment, and continuous monitoring to prevent serious cardiovascular complications associated with uncontrolled secondary hypertension.

Keywords: secondary hypertension, causes, diagnosis, treatment, endocrine disorders, renal diseases

1. Introduction

High blood pressure, or hypertension, can either be primary (essential) or secondary. Primary hypertension is the more common form, where no specific underlying cause is identified. In contrast, secondary hypertension occurs when high blood pressure is the result of another health condition. Though less common than primary hypertension, secondary hypertension is still not fully understood and often remains undiagnosed.

Secondary hypertension is more likely to affect younger individuals and those whose high blood pressure is difficult to control with standard treatments. Identifying the underlying cause of secondary hypertension is crucial, as treating the root condition can significantly reduce the risk of heart disease, stroke, and other serious health issues, improving overall quality of life [1]. As noted by Viera, secondary hypertension is a form of high blood pressure with a treatable cause [2].

The recognition of high blood pressure has evolved in recent years. In 2017, the American College of Cardiology and the American Heart Association (ACC/AHA) lowered the threshold for defining hypertension to 130/80 mmHg or higher. This is in contrast to the European guidelines (2018–2023), which define hypertension as blood pressure above 140/90 mmHg [3].

Despite treatment, many patients still struggle to control their blood pressure to below the target of 140/90 mmHg, suggesting the possibility of secondary hypertension. Sudano et al. highlight that secondary hypertension may be present in these cases, especially if blood pressure increases suddenly or becomes dangerously high, which can be a sign of an underlying condition [4].

The importance of identifying secondary hypertension cannot be exaggerated. Chronic hypertension, regardless of the cause, can lead to serious damage to vital organs, including the heart, kidneys, brain, and eyes [5]. While most patients with hypertension have primary hypertension (with no known cause), identifying secondary causes is essential because, with proper treatment, secondary hypertension can often be cured [6]. Therefore, recognizing and addressing secondary hypertension is a key step in the effective management and prevention of long-term health complications.

2. Causes of secondary hypertension

Secondary hypertension is categorized based on its underlying causes into various subgroups. These include renal hypertension (divided into renoparenchymal and renovascular), as well as endocrine-related hypertension (such as primary aldosteronism, Cushing's syndrome or disease, pheochromocytoma, and thyroid/parathyroid disorders). Other contributing factors to secondary hypertension encompass sleep-disordered breathing, aortic coarctation, pregnancy-induced hypertension (such as Hemolysis, Elevated Liver Enzymes, and Low Platelet [HELLP] syndrome), certain chemotherapeutic drugs, and treatment-resistant primary hypertension. The primary causes and their mechanisms for inducing secondary hypertension are summarized in the following sections.

2.1 Kidney and renal artery disease

The kidneys are crucial in regulating blood pressure. While arterial hypertension can cause kidney destruction, diseases affecting the kidneys and renal arteries can also lead to elevated blood pressure. Renal hypertension may result from chronic renal insufficiency (CRI) of various causes or from renal artery stenosis (RAS). Secondary forms of renal hypertension comprise glomerular disorders, such as glomerulonephritis, tubulointerstitial conditions like polycystic kidney disease, or microvascular kidney injury and renovascular blood pressure [7].

Renal artery stenosis should be considered as a potential cause of hypertension in younger individuals, particularly women with fibromuscular dysplasia, who do not have a family history of hypertension, or in older patients presenting with hypertensive crises, flash pulmonary edema (often associated with bilateral renal artery stenosis), or unexplained progressive renal function decline. The prevalence of different causes of renal artery stenosis varies with age and cardiovascular risk factors, with atherosclerotic renal artery stenosis accounting for 60–90% of cases and fibromuscular dysplasia responsible for 10–30% of cases [8].

Fibromuscular dysplasia, primarily observed in young women, should be distinguished from atherosclerotic artery stenosis, which is more prevalent in older persons [7]. It is a non-atherosclerotic, noninflammatory vascular disorder that affects the renal, iliac, subclavian, and carotid arteries. In the renal arteries, changes are typically observed in the distal segments, displaying a "string-of-beads" pattern, as well as in the segmental arteries, where there are characteristic "pearl necklace" patterns in the arterial walls.

Atherosclerotic renal artery stenosis is commonly found in older individuals with cardiovascular risk factors, including dyslipidemia, diabetes, and tobacco use. It is also prevalent in patients with atherosclerotic involvement of other vessels, such as peripheral arterial disease or coronary and cerebrovascular disease. In contrast to fibromuscular dysplasia, atherosclerotic lesions typically develop in the proximal segments of the renal arteries.

2.1.1 Pathophysiology of renal artery stenosis (renovascular disease) as a cause of secondary hypertension

According to Klabunde [9], renal artery disease can lead to the narrowing of the vessel lumen (stenosis), which reduces the pressure in the afferent arteriole and impairs renal perfusion. This triggers the kidneys to release renin, resulting in elevated levels of angiotensin II (AII) and aldosterone. These hormones raise blood volume by increasing the reabsorption of sodium and water in the kidneys, which in turn boosts cardiac output (CO) *via* the Frank-Starling mechanism. Elevated AII also causes systemic vasoconstriction, increasing systemic vascular resistance (SVR), and stimulates sympathetic activity. Chronic AII elevation further promotes cardiac and vascular hypertrophy. As a result, hypertension associated with renal artery stenosis is driven by both an increase in systemic vascular resistance and a rise in cardiac output.

2.1.2 Pathophysiology of chronic renal disease as a cause of secondary hypertension

Pathological conditions like diabetic nephropathy and glomerulonephritis can impair nephron function, reducing the kidneys' ability to excrete sodium effectively. This leads to sodium and water preservation, increased blood volume, and elevated cardiac output *via* the Frank-Starling mechanism. Additionally, renal disease may stimulate excessive renin secretion, contributing to renin-dependent hypertension. The rise in arterial pressure associated with renal dysfunction is often interpreted as a compensatory response aimed at improving renal perfusion and maintaining glomerular filtration [9].

2.2 Endocrine causes of secondary hypertension

Endocrine disorders contribute significantly to cases of secondary hypertension, with elevated blood pressure in these cases often being referred to as endocrine hypertension. The majority of these cases are due to primary aldosteronism. Other, less common causes include certain types of pheochromocytomas, Cushing's syndrome, acromegaly, and thyroid or parathyroid disorders [10]. More recently, insulinoma has also been identified as a potential cause of secondary hypertension [3].

2.2.1 Primary aldosteronism

Primary aldosteronism, also known as hyperaldosteronism, is the leading cause of secondary hypertension in middle-aged adults (ages 40–64 years) [2]. It is actually a collection of conditions, including aldosterone-producing adenomas and bilateral idiopathic hyperaldosteronism. Primary aldosteronism affects approximately 10–20% of patients with resistant hypertension, making it the most frequent cause of secondary hypertension in this age group.

Pathophysiology of primary aldosteronism as a cause of secondary hypertension.

An adrenal adenoma or adrenal hyperplasia can lead to excessive aldosterone secretion. The elevated levels of aldosterone cause the kidneys to retain sodium and water, which results in increased blood volume and higher arterial pressure. As the body tries to suppress the renin-angiotensin system, plasma renin levels are typically low. Additionally, high aldosterone levels are often associated with hypokalemia.

2.2.2 Phaeochromocytoma

Tumors that secrete excessive amounts of catecholamines are known as "phaeo-chromocytomas" or "paragangliomas," depending on their anatomical location. These lesions may occur in the adrenal glands (phaeochromocytomas) or in sympathetic ganglia found along the sympathetic chain (paragangliomas or extra-adrenal phaeo-chromocytomas). Both phaeochromocytomas and paragangliomas are rare tumors, accounting for less than 0.1% of all cases of hypertension [7].

2.2.2.1 Pathophysiology of pheochromocytoma as a cause of secondary hypertension

Catecholamine-secreting tumors in the adrenal medulla can result in extremely high levels of circulating catecholamines, including both epinephrine and nor-epinephrine. The elevated catecholamine levels induce systemic vasoconstriction through alpha-adrenoceptors and enhance cardiac activity *via* beta-adrenoceptors, with cardiac stimulation leading to a substantial increase in arterial pressure. Although blood pressure rises, tachycardia arises due to the direct influence of catecholamines on the heart and vasculature. Overstimulation of β-adrenoceptors in the heart often leads to the development of arrhythmias.

2.2.3 Cushing's syndrome

Cushing's syndrome, also referred to as glucocorticoid excess syndrome, is another potential cause of secondary hypertension. Although an excess of glucocorticoids contributes to blood pressure regulation, arterial hypertension is seldom the primary clinical manifestation in patients with Cushing's syndrome.

2.2.3.1 Pathophysiology of Cushing's syndrome as a cause of secondary hypertension

In Cushing's syndrome (CS), hypertension develops due to multiple pathophysi-ological mechanisms that contribute to increased plasma volume, peripheral vascular resistance, and cardiac output. Glucocorticoids may also affect blood pressure control by acting on the central nervous system, where they activate both glucocorticoid and mineralocorticoid receptors (MR). As a result, glucocorticoids lead to changes that elevate cardiac output, total peripheral resistance, and renovascular resistance [11], which contributes to persistent hypertension. Additionally, insulin resistance and sleep apnea seem to be involved in the development of hypertension in CS.

2.2.4 Thyroid and parathyroid diseases

Dysregulation of thyroid and parathyroid function are reversible causes of secondary hypertension [12]. Thyroid disorders lead to various hemodynamic changes that contribute to elevated blood pressure through their effects on endothelial function, vascular reactivity, renal hemodynamics, and the renin-angiotensin system.

In hyperthyroidism, the increased endothelial responsiveness is a result of shear stress from the hyperdynamic circulation, which helps lower vascular resistance. On the other hand, hypothyroidism leads to a marked reduction in sensitivity to sympathetic agonists, resulting in higher peripheral vascular resistance and arterial stiffness.

Sporadic primary hyperparathyroidism is an endocrine disorder often characterized by persistent fasting hypercalcemia, caused by the autonomous overproduction of parathyroid hormone due to parathyroid adenoma or hyperplasia (hypercalcemic primary hyperparathyroidism). Primary hyperparathyroidism is associated with a higher risk of arterial hypertension, with studies showing that 40–65% of patients with this condition also have high blood pressure [13]. Notably, hypertensive patients with primary hyperparathyroidism have a higher mortality rate compared to those who are normotensive.

2.2.4.1 Pathophysiology of hyper or hypothyroidism as a cause of secondary hypertension

Increased thyroxine levels lead to higher blood volume by activating the renin-angiotensin-aldosterone system, along with an elevated heart rate and enhanced ventricular contractility. Conversely, low thyroxine levels (hypothyroidism) reduce tissue metabolism, which may decrease the production of vasodilatory metabolites and the endothelial production of nitric oxide, resulting in vasoconstriction and elevated arterial pressure. Additionally, there is an increase in arterial stiffness, or reduced arterial compliance.

2.2.5 Insulinoma

Pancreatic insulinomas are uncommon, usually benign, small neuroendocrine tumors, approximated to affect 1–4 people per million per year. The typical age of individuals affected is about 47 years, and these tumors are more common in women than in men (with a ratio of 1.4:1). These tumors are characterized by chronic, sustained hyperinsulinemia, which leads to recurrent hypoglycemia [3]. Evidence suggests that hyperinsulinemia and insulin resistance may be early factors in the development of secondary hypertension. There are several mechanisms through which pancreatic insulinomas can cause secondary hypertension. First, severe hypoglycemia caused by the insulinoma can stimulate the release of catecholamines, resulting in paroxysmal hypertension due to the activation of the sympathoadrenal system. Second, insulin may enhance sodium retention in the kidneys, especially in the distal nephron, and cause changes in the vascular system, both of which contribute to elevated blood pressure [14].

2.3 Other causes of secondary hypertension

2.3.1 Aortic coarctation

Coarctation of the aorta is a congenital condition in which the aorta, the main artery leaving the left side of the heart, becomes narrowed, restricting normal blood flow and raising blood pressure. This narrowing most commonly occurs just below the left subclavian artery in the aortic arch. The obstruction reduces blood pressure in the lower body while raising pressure in the head and upper limbs. The drop in systemic arterial pressure triggers the renin-angiotensin-aldosterone system, leading to an increase in blood volume, which further elevates blood pressure in the upper parts of the body and may largely offset the reduction in pressure in the lower parts of the body. Coarctation is easily diagnosed by comparing blood pressure readings in the upper and lower limbs. Typically, these pressures are comparable, but in coarctation, blood pressure in the upper limbs is often significantly higher than in the lower limbs. Since this condition is persistent, baroreceptors become less responsive, resulting in persistent high blood pressure in the upper body due to increased cardiac output to those areas [9].

2.3.2 Sleep-disordered breathing/sleep apnea

Sleep apnea is a condition in which individuals experience repeated episodes of breathing cessation for brief periods (10–30 seconds) during sleep. While it is commonly linked to obesity, it can also result from other factors, such as airway obstruction or central nervous system disorders. Individuals with sleep apnea are more likely to develop elevated blood pressure. This elevated blood pressure may be caused by the stimulation of the sympathetic nervous system and hormonal changes resulting from recurring episodes of apnea-induced hypoxia and hypercapnia, as well as the stress associated with disrupted sleep.

2.3.3 Pregnancy-induced secondary hypertension (preeclampsia/HELLP syndrome)

Pregnancy-induced secondary hypertension refers to a spectrum of hypertensive disorders unique to pregnancy, with preeclampsia and Hemolysis, Elevated Liver Enzymes, and Low Platelet (HELLP) syndrome being the most severe forms. These conditions present significant risks to maternal and fetal health, arising from complex interactions between the cardiovascular, endocrine, and immune systems during pregnancy.

In a normal pregnancy, systemic vascular resistance decreases, and blood volume expands to support the growing fetus, facilitated by hormonal and vascular adaptations. However, in preeclampsia and HELLP syndrome, these mechanisms are disrupted due to abnormal placental development. Poor trophoblast invasion leads to insufficient remodeling of maternal spiral arteries, resulting in impaired placental perfusion and chronic hypoxia. In response, the placenta releases a surge of antiangiogenic factors such as soluble fms-like tyrosine kinase-1 (sFlt-1) and soluble endoglin (sEng), which counteract vascular endothelial growth factor (VEGF) and transforming growth factor-beta (TGF-β). This imbalance causes widespread endothelial dysfunction, increased systemic vascular resistance, and hypertension.

Preeclampsia, diagnosed after 20 weeks of gestation, is marked by new-onset hypertension, often accompanied by proteinuria or evidence of organ damage.

HELLP syndrome, considered a severe variant of preeclampsia, involves systemic inflammation, intravascular hemolysis, and microvascular injury. Hepatic dysfunction and platelet consumption are key features, reflecting the multiorgan impact of the condition.

The pathophysiology of these disorders extends beyond vascular changes to include immune dysregulation and oxidative stress. Altered maternal immune responses, heightened sensitivity to angiotensin II, and an imbalance in pro- and anti-inflammatory cytokines exacerbate endothelial injury and vasoconstriction. Hemodynamic changes, including increased cardiac output *via* the Frank-Starling mechanism, further strain the maternal circulatory system, contributing to elevated blood pressure.

Understanding the physiology underlying pregnancy-induced secondary hypertension is essential for early detection and management, ultimately aiming to reduce the burden of maternal and neonatal complications.

HELLP syndrome is a variant of preeclampsia. In preeclampsia, atypical changes in the placental blood vessels during the second trimester occur, during which the second phase of trophoblastic invasion into the decidua takes place, resulting in poor blood flow to the placenta. This lack of oxygen in the placenta causes it to release various substances, including soluble vascular endothelial growth factor receptor-1 (sVEGFR-1), which binds to vascular endothelial growth factor (VEGF) and placental growth factor (PGF). This binding prevents VEGF and PGF from attaching to endothelial cell receptors, resulting in endothelial dysfunction and placental damage. As a result, hypertension, proteinuria, and heightened platelet activation and aggregation occur. Additionally, the stimulation of the coagulation process causes platelet depletion as they stick to damaged and activated blood vessel linings. Microangiopathic hemolysis also takes place as red blood cells are broken apart while moving through capillaries obstructed by platelet-fibrin clots. This results in multiorgan microvascular injury and hepatic necrosis, which contributes to liver dysfunction and the development of HELLP syndrome [15–19]. **Figure 1** presents a summary of causes of secondary hypertension.

Common causes of secondary hypertension usually vary with age [2]. The summary of common causes of secondary hypertension according to age groups is shown in **Table 1** below.

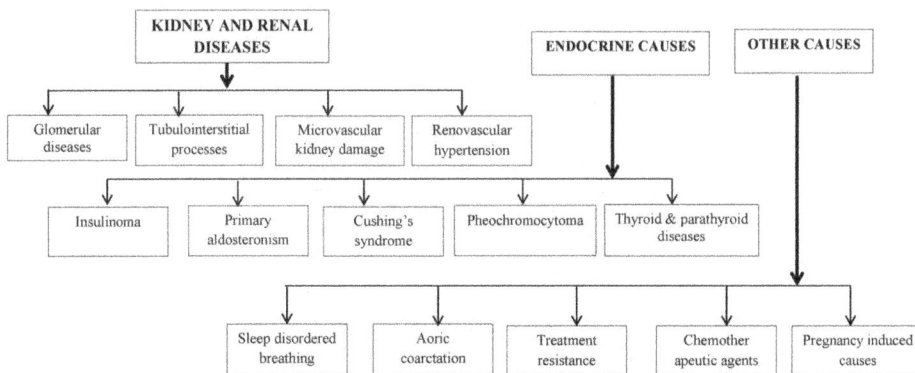

Figure 1.
Causes of secondary hypertension.

Age group	Most common etiologies
Children (birth-12 years)	Renal parenchymal disease; coarctation of the aorta
Adolescents (12–18 years)	Renal parenchymal disease; coarctation of the aorta
Young adults (19–39 years)	thyroid dysfunction; fibromuscular dysplasia; renal parenchymal disease
Middle-aged adults (40–64 years)	Primary aldosteronism; obstructive sleep apnea; thyroid dysfunction; Cushing's syndrome; pheochromocytoma
Older adults (65 years and older)	Atherosclerotic renal artery stenosis; renal diseases/renal failure; Hypothyroidism

Source: Ref. [2].

Table 1.
Common causes of secondary hypertension according to age.

3. Diagnostic tests of secondary hypertension

Imaging plays a critical role in diagnosing the underlying causes of hypertension, evaluating its cardiovascular complications, and understanding the disease's pathophysiology. Cardiovascular magnetic resonance (CMR) is particularly effective as it provides accurate, reproducible measurements of ventricular volumes, mass, function, and hemodynamics while also allowing for unique tissue characterization, such as identifying diffuse and focal fibrosis. Moreover, CMR is highly suitable for identifying common secondary causes of hypertension.

CMR offers a thorough evaluation of hypertensive cardiovascular disease. Within an hour, precise and consistent measurements of the ventricles and aorta can be obtained. This includes assessing the physiological consequences of hypertension and generating quantitative data that are valuable for patient follow-up. Simultaneously, the study can rule out several secondary hypertension causes. In terms of prognostic insights, advancements in T1 mapping sequences for quantifying myocardial fibrosis may significantly aid in risk assessment for hypertensive heart disease [5].

Contrast agents are used in magnetic resonance imaging (MRI) to enhance the visibility of detailed organ structures. Gadolinium-based contrast agents (GBCAs) have been in use since 1988, improving MRI diagnostics and patient follow-up by increasing signal intensity and reducing proton relaxation time. However, recent studies have highlighted concerns over gadolinium accumulation in various organs due to the release of free gadolinium, which has raised safety issues. These studies focus on the impact of gadolinium retention in organs like the brain and bones, with associated conditions including nephrogenic systemic fibrosis (NSF) and gadolinium deposition disease (GDD). Research continues to develop non-gadolinium-based agents and next-generation gadolinium agents for safer applications in MRI [20].

Thyroid hormones influence cardiac output and systemic vascular resistance, which subsequently impact blood pressure. Hypothyroidism may result in increased diastolic blood pressure, while hyperthyroidism often causes isolated systolic blood pressure elevation, leading to a widened pulse pressure. Although hypothyroidism is a common secondary cause of hypertension in younger adults, its prevalence increases with age, peaking in the 60s. In contrast, hyperthyroidism is more commonly linked to elevated blood pressure in individuals aged 20–50 years. Given thyroid dysfunction's prevalence across age groups, it is recommended to test for thyroid-stimulating hormone (TSH) if symptoms suggest its involvement. TSH is a sensitive marker for diagnosing both conditions [2].

Zhang et al. [21] proposed a simple, effective method to predict renal artery stenosis (RAS) of 70% or greater using peak systolic velocity (PSV) and PSV ratios obtained through basic duplex ultrasound (DUS). This technique has the potential to detect severe RAS in most medical facilities, particularly in primary care settings, and provides a reliable basis for selecting candidates for angiography or revascularization.

The aldosterone-to-renin ratio (ARR) remains the standard screening test for primary aldosteronism (PA). Due to its low reproducibility, repeat testing is recommended when results conflict with clinical observations. Taiwan's Task Force on PA recommends using plasma renin activity (PRA) to calculate ARR instead of direct renin concentration (DRC), aligning with international guidelines and most studies [22].

Polysomnography (PSG) is the gold standard for diagnosing obstructive sleep apnea (OSA). However, due to its cost, complexity, and resource requirements, alternative methods have been explored. Studies suggest that overnight pulse oximetry can be a reliable diagnostic tool for suspected sleep apnea-hypopnea syndrome (SAHS), with sensitivity, specificity, and accuracy improving with the severity of the condition [23].

Pheochromocytoma and paraganglioma (PPGL) diagnoses rely on biochemical confirmation of excessive catecholamines in urine and plasma. New advancements allow for measuring urinary free metanephrines, providing greater reliability compared to older biochemical methods, especially in Asian populations [24].

Finally, research by Carton revealed limitations in using the 1 mg-dexamethasone suppression test (1 mg-DST) for women on oral contraceptives due to its low specificity. The two-day dexamethasone suppression test (2d-DST) showed better specificity and accuracy. It may be preferable in cases where late-night salivary cortisol tests are unavailable, particularly if the initial cortisol concentration is below 900 nmol/L [25]. The typical signs and symptoms of some secondary hypertension causes and suggested diagnostic tests are summarized in **Table 2**.

Signs/symptoms	Possible secondary hypertension cause	Diagnostic test options
Arm to leg systolic blood pressure difference > 20 mm Hg Delayed or absent femoral pulses, Murmur	Coarctation of the aorta	Magnetic resonance imaging (adults) Transthoracic echocardiography (children)
Increase in serum creatinine concentration (≥ 0.5–1 mg per dL [44.20–88.40 μmol per L]) after starting angiotensin-converting enzyme inhibitor or angiotensin receptor blocker Renal bruit	Renal artery stenosis	Computed tomography angiography Doppler ultrasonography of renal arteries Magnetic resonance imaging with gadolinium contrast media
Bradycardia/tachycardia Cold/heat intolerance Constipation/diarrhea Irregular, heavy, or absent menstrual cycle	Thyroid disorders	Thyroid-stimulating hormone

Signs/symptoms	Possible secondary hypertension cause	Diagnostic test options
Hypokalemia	Aldosteronism	Renin and aldosterone levels to calculate the aldosterone/renin ratio
Apneic events during sleep Daytime sleepiness Snoring	Obstructive sleep apnea	Polysomnography (sleep study) sleep apnea clinical score with nighttime pulse oximetry
Flushing Headaches Labile blood pressures Orthostatic hypotension Palpitations Sweating Syncope	Pheochromocytoma	24-hour urinary fractionated metanephrines Plasma free metanephrines
Buffalo hump Central obesity Moon facies Striae	Cushing's syndrome	24-hour urinary cortisol Late-night salivary cortisol Low-dose dexamethasone suppression

Table 2.
Signs and symptoms that suggest specific causes and suggested diagnostic tests of secondary hypertension.

4. Treatment and prognosis of secondary hypertension

The management of secondary hypertension involves treating the underlying cause while optimizing blood pressure control to prevent complications. The therapeutic approach varies depending on the etiology and may include lifestyle modifications, pharmacological therapy, and interventional or surgical procedures.

4.1 Lifestyle modifications

Lifestyle changes play a crucial role in blood pressure management. Patients are advised to adopt the Dietary Approaches to Stop Hypertension (DASH) diet, which emphasizes the consumption of fruits, vegetables, whole grains, and low-fat dairy while reducing sodium intake [26]. Weight loss is essential, particularly in obesity-related hypertension, as even modest reductions in body weight can significantly lower blood pressure [27]. Regular aerobic exercise, such as brisk walking for at least 30 minutes daily, is recommended. Additionally, reducing alcohol intake and smoking cessation are critical in improving cardiovascular outcomes [28].

4.2 Pharmacological therapy

Targeted pharmacologic treatment depends on the underlying cause of hypertension. Diuretics, such as spironolactone, are effective in primary aldosteronism, whereas beta-blockers, like propranolol, are used in pheochromocytoma to control catecholamine surges [29]. Calcium channel blockers (e.g., amlodipine) are preferred in renovascular hypertension, although angiotensin-converting enzyme (ACE) inhibitors or angiotensin receptor blockers (ARBs) should be used cautiously in bilateral renal artery stenosis due to the risk of renal function deterioration [30].

4.3 Surgical and interventional approaches

For cases where pharmacologic management is insufficient, surgical or interventional procedures may be required. Renal artery stenosis may necessitate angioplasty or stenting, particularly in cases of refractory hypertension or declining renal function [31]. Adrenalectomy is the definitive treatment for pheochromocytoma or aldosterone-producing adenomas, leading to potential cure or significant blood pressure reduction [32]. In cases of hypothyroidism-induced hypertension, thyroid hormone replacement therapy is essential for normalization of blood pressure [33]. Patients with end-stage renal disease (ESRD) secondary to hypertension may require dialysis or renal transplantation to control blood pressure and prevent further complications [34].

5. Prognosis

The prognosis of secondary hypertension is largely determined by the reversibility of the underlying condition, the efficacy of treatment, and the presence of target organ damage. Conditions such as pheochromocytoma, primary aldosteronism, and renovascular hypertension may be curable with appropriate intervention, leading to complete resolution or significant improvement in blood pressure control [35]. In contrast, chronic kidney disease (CKD), endocrine disorders, and coexisting cardiovascular conditions often require lifelong management to prevent disease progression [36].

Patients with uncontrolled or poorly managed secondary hypertension are at increased risk of complications, including myocardial infarction, stroke, heart failure, and kidney failure. Hypertensive emergencies, if left untreated, can lead to irreversible organ damage [37]. However, early diagnosis and effective treatment significantly improve long-term outcomes, reducing cardiovascular morbidity and mortality. Regular follow-up, adherence to medications, and blood pressure monitoring are essential, particularly for patients with chronic conditions such as CKD or endocrine hypertension [38].

Author details

Titus F. Msoka
KCMC University, Moshi, Tanzania

*Address all correspondence to: titus.msoka@kcmcu.ac.tz

IntechOpen

References

[1] Sarathy H, Salman LA, Lee C, Cohen JB. Evaluation and Management of Secondary Hypertension. The Medical Clinics of North America. 2022;**106**(2):269-283. DOI: 10.1016/j.mcna.2021.11.004

[2] Viera AJ, Neutze DM. Diagnosis of secondary hypertension: An age-based approach. American Family Physician. 2010;**82**(12):1471-1478

[3] Mijalkovic M, Sacic D. A new potential cause of secondary hypertension. Cardiovascular Medicine. 2024;**11**:1458089. DOI: 10.3389/fcvm.2024.1458089

[4] Sudano I, Suter P, Beuschlein F. Secondary hypertension as a cause of treatment resistance. Blood Pressure. 2023;**32**(1):2224898. DOI: 10.1080/08037051.2023.2224898

[5] Maceira AM, Mohiaddin RH. Cardiovascular magnetic resonance in systemic hypertension. Journal of Cardiovascular Magnetic Resonance. 2012;**14**:28

[6] Freihage JH, Nanjundappa A, Dieter RS. Secondary hypertension: Etiology and mechanism of disease. Therapy. 2008;**5**(6):787-790. DOI: 10.2217/14750708.5.6.787

[7] Sudano I, Beuschlein F, Lüscher TF. Secondary causes of hypertension. In: Camm AJ, editor. The ESC Textbook of Cardiovascular Medicine. 3rd ed. Oxford, UK: Publisher Oxford University Press; 2018. pp. 1-10

[8] Safian RD, Textor SC. Renal-artery stenosis. The New England Journal of Medicine. 2001;**344**(6):431-442. DOI: 10.1056/NEJM200102083440607

[9] Klabunde RE. Cardiovascular Physiology Concepts. 3rd ed. Philadelphia, Pennsylvania, USA: Publisher Wolters Kluwer; 2021

[10] Sudano I, Suter P, Beuschlein F. Secondary hypertension as a cause of treatment resistance. Blood Pressure. 2023;**32**:1. DOI: 10.1080/08037051.2023.2224898

[11] Muiesan ML, Lupia M, Salvetti M, Grigoletto C, Sonino N, Boscaro M, et al. Left ventricular structural and functional characteristics in Cushing's syndrome. Journal of the American College of Cardiology. 2003;**41**:2275-2279

[12] Mazza A, Beltramello G, Armigliato M, et al. Arterial hypertension and thyroid disorders: What is important to know in clinical practice? Annales d'Endocrinologie. 2011;**72**(4):296-303. DOI: 10.1016/j.ando.2011.05.004

[13] Schiffl H, Lang SM. Hypertension secondary to PHPT: Cause or coincidence? International Journal of Endocrinology. 2011;**2011**:974647. DOI: 10.1155/2011/974647

[14] Mijalkovic M, Sacic D, Pajovic S. A rare case of pancreatic insulinoma, sleep apnea, and hypertension. Cardiology Research and Cardiovascular Medicine. 2024;**9**:243. DOI: 10.29011/2575-7083.100243

[15] Rahman TM, Wendon J. Severe hepatic dysfunction in pregnancy. The Quarterly Journal of Medicine. 2002;**95**:343

[16] Knerr I, Beinder E, Rascher W. Syncytin, a novel human endogenous retroviral gene in human placenta:

Evidence for its dysregulation in preeclampsia and HELLP syndrome. American Journal of Obstetrics and Gynecology. 2002;**186**:210

[17] Levine RJ, Maynard SE, Qian C, et al. Circulating angiogenic factors and the risk of preeclampsia. The New England Journal of Medicine. 2004;**350**:672

[18] Mutter WP, Karumanchi SA. Molecular mechanisms of preeclampsia. Microvascular Research. 2008;**75**:1

[19] Widmer M, Villar J, Beniani A, et al. Mapping the theories of preeclampsia and the role of angiogenic factors: A systematic review. Obstet Gynecol 109:168, 2007. Obstetrics and Gynecology. 2007;**109**:168

[20] Iyad N, Ahmad MS, Alkhatib SG, Hjouj M. Gadolinium contrast agents: Challenges and opportunities of a multidisciplinary approach-literature review. European Journal of Radiology (London, UK: Elsevier Ltd.). DOI: 10.1016/j.ejro.2023.100503

[21] Zhang Y, Wang Y, Na M, Li Y, Li Y, Ren J. Application of simple ultrasound Doppler hemodynamic parameters in the diagnosis of severe renal artery stenosis in routine clinical practice. Quantitative Imaging in Medicine and Surgery. 2023;**13**(12):8042-8052. DOI: 10.21037/qims-23-605

[22] Lin C-H, Lin C-H, Chung M-C, Hung C-S, Fe TF-Y, Er LK, et al. Aldosterone-to-renin ratio (ARR) as a screening tool for primary aldosteronism (PA). Journal of the Formosan Medical Association (Taiwan). 2024;**123**:598-S103. DOI: 10.1016/j.jfma.2023.04.019

[23] Sullman L, Shalabi N, Saad A. Validity of overnight pulse oximetry as a screening tool of obstructive sleep apnea. European Respiratory Journal. 2016;**48**(Suppl 60):PA2316. DOI: 10.1183/13993003.congress-2016. PA2316

[24] Ahn J, Park JY, Kim G, Jin S-M, Hur KY, Lee S-Y, et al. Urinary free metanephrines for diagnosis of pheochromocytoma and paraganglioma. Endocrinology and Metabolism. 2021;**36**:697-701. DOI: 10.3803/EnM.2020.925

[25] Carton T, Mathieu E, Wolff F, Bouziotis J, Corvilain B, Driessens N. Two-day low-dose dexamethasone suppression test more accurate than overnight 1-mg in women taking oral contraceptive. Endocrinology, Diabetes and Metabolism. 2021;**4**(3):e00255. DOI: 10.1002/edm2.255

[26] Whelton PK, Carey RM, Aronow WS, Casey DE, Collins KJ, Himmelfarb CD, et al. ACC/AHA/AAPA/ABC/ACPM/AGS/APhA/ASH/ASPC/NMA/PCNA guideline for the prevention, detection, evaluation, and management of high blood pressure in adults: A report of the American College of Cardiology/American Heart Association task force on clinical practice guidelines. Journal of the American College of Cardiology. 2018;**71**(19):e127-e248

[27] Williams B, Mancia G, Spiering W, Agabiti Rosei E, Azizi M, Burnier M, et al. ESC/ESH guidelines for the management of arterial hypertension. European Heart Journal. 2018;**39**(33):3021-3104

[28] Fuchs FD, Whelton PK. High blood pressure and cardiovascular disease. Hypertension. 2020;**75**(2):285-292

[29] Funder JW, Carey RM, Mantero F, Murad MH, Reincke M, Shibata H, et al. The management of primary aldosteronism: Case detection, diagnosis,

and treatment: An endocrine society clinical practice guideline. The Journal of Clinical Endocrinology and Metabolism. 2016;**101**(5):1889-1916

[30] Rossi GP, Bisogni V, Rossitto G, Maiolino G, Cesari M, Zhu R, et al. Practice recommendations for diagnosis and treatment of the most common forms of secondary hypertension. High Blood Pressure and Cardiovascular Prevention. 2020;**27**:547-560. DOI: 10.1007/s40292-020-00415-9

[31] Textor SC. Atherosclerotic renal artery stenosis: Overtreated but still undertreated? Journal of the American Society of Nephrology. 2008;**4**:656-659. DOI: 10.1681/ ASN.2007111204

[32] Young WF Jr. Primary aldosteronism: A common and curable form of hypertension. Cardiology in Review. 1999;**7**(4):207-214

[33] Cappola AR, Desai AS, Medici M, Cooper LS, Egan D, Sopko G, et al. The thyroid and cardiovascular disease: A research agenda for enhancing knowledge, prevention, and treatment. Circulation. 2019;**139**(25):2892-2909. DOI: 10.1161

[34] Ku E, Lee BJ, Wei J, Weir MR. Hypertension in CKD: Core curriculum 2019. American Journal of Kidney Diseases. 2019;**74**(1):120-131. DOI: 10.1053/j.ajkd.2018.12.044

[35] Mazza A, Armigliato M, Cristina Marzola M, Schiavon L, Montemurro D, Vescovo G, et al. Anti-hypertensive treatment in pheochromocytoma and paraganglioma: Current management and therapeutic features. Endocrine. 2014;**45**(3):469-478. DOI: 10.1007/ s12020-013-0007-y

[36] Vallianou NF, Mitesh S, Gkogkou A, Geladari E. Chronic kidney disease and cardiovascular disease: Is there any relationship? Current Cardiology Reviews. 2019;**15**:55-63. DOI: 10.2174/157 3403X14666180711124825

[37] Calhoun DA, Booth JN, Oparil S, Irvin MR, Shimbo D, Lackland DT, et al. Refractory hypertension: Determination of prevalence, risk factors and comorbidities in a large. Population-Based Cohort. Hypertension. 2014;**63**(3):451-458. DOI: 10.1161/ HYPERTENSIONAHA.113.02026

[38] Hebert SA, Ibrahim HN. Hypertension management in patients with chronic kidney disease. Journal of Cardiovascular Medicine. 2022;**18**(4): 41-49. DOI: 10.14797/m dcvj.1119

Chapter 6

Hypertension Control: The Effect of Dietary Patterns and Lifestyle

Othman Beni Yonis

Abstract

Hypertension is one of the most important and serious global health diseases. The prevalence rate is high and increasing (31.1% of adults worldwide). Up to 1.5 billion people will suffer hypertension by 2025; it is also one of the main risk factors for coronary artery disease, heart failure, cerebrovascular, renal, eye, and peripheral vascular diseases. According to the World Heart Federation, the mortality from hypertension complications is around 10 million each year. The morbidity and mortality from hypertension are preventable, and the risk to develop hypertension and hypertension complications is lowered significantly by controlling blood pressure to below the target level. However, uncontrolled hypertension is still a major health concern globally. Only about half of hypertension patients have had their blood pressure brought down to below the recommended limit, which is 140/90 mmHg. Adopting and maintaining a healthy lifestyle plays a major role in hypertension prevention and control. Morbidity and mortality rates secondary to hypertension are also improved. In conclusion, besides adherence and commitment to antihypertension medications, dietary patterns including low salt diet, weight control, exercise and physical activity, stress management, and avoiding tobacco and alcohol are all recommended to prevent, treat, and minimize morbidity and mortality associated with hypertension. In this chapter, we will discuss the effect of dietary patterns and other lifestyle interventions on blood pressure control.

Keywords: hypertension control, lifestyle and hypertension, diet and hypertension, salt and hypertension, anxiety and hypertension, stress and hypertension, physical activity and hypertension, weight and hypertension

1. Introduction

Hypertension is defined as a sustained elevation of systemic arterial blood pressure, most commonly defined as systolic blood pressure ≥ 140 mmHg or diastolic blood pressure ≥ 90 mmHg. It affects approximately 31% of the global adult population and is characterized by a rising prevalence [1, 2]. The mortality rate of hypertension is about 13% [3].

The morbidity and mortality from hypertension are preventable. The risk to develop hypertension and hypertension complications is lowered significantly by controlling blood pressure (BP). With control, the risk of heart failure is reduced by over 50%, stroke by 30%, and myocardial infarction by 25% [3].

However, uncontrolled hypertension is still a major health concern. Globally, only about half of hypertension patients have had their BP brought down to below the recommended limit, which is 140/90 mmHg [4].

Studies conducted on hypertension control worldwide showed varying rates of control. The National Health and Nutrition Examination Survey (NHANES) statistics in the United States indicated that although hypertension control rates had improved, they were still low [5]. According to Olives et al., the median rates for controlling hypertension in the United States were 57.7% for males and 57.1% for women, with the highest rates observed in white men and black women [4].

The disparity in hypertension control between industrialized and developing countries was examined in 35 countries as part of a systematic review. North America had the highest control rate (24.9%) among men, while northern and central Asia had the lowest (5.7%). Nonetheless, among women, it was highest in South and Central America (33.2%) and lowest in North Europe (10%) [6].

Many studies and reviews (see below) investigated the role of nonpharmacological strategies to prevent, treat, and control hypertension. In this review we will discuss these strategies and explore the role of each factor separately.

2. Discussion

2.1 The effect of lifestyle and dietary patterns on blood pressure control

Many studies have examined the relationship between dietary lifestyle habits and controlling high BP. As for salt, consuming larger amounts of dietary salt is clearly linked to high BP and other cardiovascular diseases. On the other hand, reducing salt intake can lead to a decrease in BP among hypertension patients as well as normal individuals.

This conclusion was reached by a meta-analysis (a method for systematically combining pertinent qualitative and quantitative study data), which showed that reducing salt intake can lower BP by an average of 3.4/1.5 mmHg, with larger reductions observed in individuals with higher baseline BP levels [7, 8].

Another study (the INTERSALT study) also highlighted the importance of salt intake on BP and stated that reducing salt consumption can ameliorate age-related hypertension [9]. Moreover, a systematic review found that long-term salt reduction is effective in lowering BP [10].

Conversely, a high-sodium diet, such as those found in the Western diet (characterized by low intakes of fruits, vegetables, whole grains, pasture-raised animal products, fish, nuts, and seeds and a high consumption of prepackaged foods, refined grains, red meat, processed meat, high-sugar drinks, candy and sweets, fried foods, butter and other high-fat dairy products, eggs, potatoes, corn, and high-fructose corn syrup) [11] has been linked to increased BP and cardiovascular diseases [12, 13].

A systematic review focused on a substitute for salt, which often replaces sodium with potassium, indicated that this substitution can lead to significant reduction in BP, particularly when used consistently over long period of time [14, 15].

Regarding other dietary patterns, consuming more fruits and vegetables and eating a low-fat diet were found to be associated with better BP control [16]. The Dietary Approaches to Stop Hypertension (DASH) eating plan or the DASH diet promoted by the U.S.-based National Heart, Lung, and Blood Institute is a dietary plan recommended for hypertensive patients and normal people to treat and prevent hypertension; it is based on eating food that is low in saturated fat, total fat, cholesterol, and sodium and high in potassium, calcium, magnesium, fiber, and protein.

The plan advises hypertensive patients to eat vegetables, fruits, and whole grains, including fat-free or low-fat dairy products, fish, poultry, beans, nuts, and vegetable oils, and to limit consuming foods that are high in saturated fat, such as fatty meats, full-fat dairy products, coconut, palm kernel, and palm oils, as well as sugar-sweetened beverages and sweets.

Olive oil and the Mediterranean (a plant-based diet, focusing on unprocessed cereals, legumes, vegetables, and fruits, moderate consumption of fish, dairy products like cheese and yogurt, and a low amount of red meat), have been found to reduce cardiovascular disease risk and BP [17].

Garlic supplements were shown to improve blood pressure control in hypertensive patients in a meta-analysis [18], but dark chocolate, which had been claimed to lower BP, was found to have no effects on it in a randomized, controlled, cross-over trial [19].

In conclusion, hypertension control and subsequent cardiovascular diseases are greatly influenced by dietary patterns: a diet that is low in salt and fat and rich in fruits and vegetables. Using salt substitutes (potassium chloride instead of sodium chloride) can further enhance the management of high BP.

2.2 Effect of exercise and physical activity on hypertension control

There is strong scientific evidence to support the effect of exercise and physical activity on BP control. Aerobic exercises and resistance training have been shown to lower BP and improve cardiovascular health. Brisk walking, jogging, or cycling, have been consistently associated with significant reductions in systolic and diastolic BP [20–23].

A systematic review showed that aerobic exercise can lead to an average reduction of 11 mmHg in systolic BP and 8 mmHg in diastolic BP among hypertensive patients [24].

Another study on resistant hypertension demonstrated that regular aerobic exercise effectively lowers BP, even in patients who are otherwise unresponsive to traditional antihypertensive therapies. The study stated that practicing regular aerobic exercise can serve as a critical adjunct to pharmacological therapy in lowering BP [25].

Resistance exercises can also lead to reductions in BP through improved vascular function, increased nitric oxide production, and enhanced muscle mass, which collectively contribute to better cardiovascular health [26].

Furthermore, the psychological benefits of physical activity cannot be ignored. Exercise has been shown to improve stress and anxiety, which are known to contribute to high BP. Regular physical activity promotes relaxation and improves overall well-being, further supporting its role in hypertension management [27].

Duration and intensity of exercise are also important. Moderate-intensity exercise, such as brisk walking for at least 150 minutes per week, is recommended for optimal benefits [28].

In summary, strong evidence supports the role of exercise and physical activity for controlling high BP, improving cardiovascular health and quality of life. Therefore, incorporating physical activity into daily routines is essential for individuals seeking to manage hypertension.

2.3 Effect of weight reduction on hypertension control

Maintaining an optimal body weight, as measured by the body mass index (BMI) of 18.5–24.9, plays a significant role in managing hypertension. Numerous studies have shown that even modest weight loss can lead to substantial improvements in BP readings [29, 30].

Weight loss improves BP by decreasing sympathetic nervous system activity, improving endothelial function, and decreasing circulating levels of inflammatory markers, factors known to contribute to lower BP [30, 31].

The more weight reduction, the more the drop in blood pressure. Each 1 kg of weight lost is associated with a reduction of approximately 1 mmHg in both systolic and diastolic BP [32, 33].

Weight reduction is also associated with improving other cardiovascular risk factors, particularly triglycerides and glucose levels [34].

Bariatric surgery is another intervention that has been studied for its effects on lowering blood pressure; significant weight loss after the surgery can even result in remission of hypertension in many patients [29].

Besides, weight loss can enhance the effectiveness of antihypertensive medications the patient is taking, allowing for fewer medications and lower doses to achieve the control [31, 35].

Moreover, the psychological gains associated with weight loss, like increased self-efficacy and improved mood, can further support adherence to lifestyle modifications that promote long-term BP control [30, 36].

In summary, weight reduction—even modest—is a strong and recommended intervention in the management of hypertension and cardiovascular health. In most cases, weight reduction is accompanied by physical activity and healthy diet, factors that are all essential components for hypertension control.

2.4 Effect of alcohol and cigarette smoking on hypertension control

Alcohol and cigarette smoking have significant adverse effects on BP, making it more difficult to control hypertension.

According to the American College of Cardiology (ACC) and the American Heart Association (AHA), both smoking and alcohol consumption are major modifiable risk factors for hypertension. These organizations recommend quitting smoking and limiting alcohol intake as part of a comprehensive strategy to manage and prevent high BP.

Alcohol intake—even moderate amounts—leads to an immediate increase in blood pressure, This is due to alcohol's impact on the autonomic nervous system, vasoconstriction, and increased heart rate. This effect may persist for several hours after consumption.

According to the AHA, alcohol consumption is a direct cause of hypertension and can impair the body's ability to regulate BP, leading to persistent high BP.

A systematic review and meta-analysis showed that reducing alcohol intake lowers BP in a dose-dependent manner with an apparent threshold effect. For people who drink more than two drinks per day, a reduction in alcohol intake was associated with greater BP reduction [37].

Regarding tobacco smoking, smoking immediately increases diastolic blood pressure and the mean arterial BP [38]. The elevated nicotine levels in the blood mediate an increase of sympathetic nervous system activities and release of epinephrine, norepinephrine, and vasopressin hormones [39–41].

A Mendelian randomization meta-analysis supports a causal association of smoking heaviness with higher level of resting heart rate, but not with BP [42]. The American Cardiac College and American Heart Association 2019 ACC/AHA Guideline on the Primary Prevention of Cardiovascular Disease strongly advised hypertensive and normal individuals to quit tobacco smoking.

In conclusion, alcohol and tobacco smoking significantly increase the risk of cardiovascular disease and worsen hypertension control. Evidence-based guidelines strongly recommend reducing alcohol intake and quitting smoking as essential steps in controlling and preventing hypertension.

2.5 Effect of anxiety and psychosocial stress on hypertension control

Chronic anxiety and psychosocial stress play a significant role in hypertension, Prolonged exposure to stress can cause BP to remain elevated, increasing the risk of hypertension. There are many suggested ways to manage stress and reduce its impact on BP such as exercise, relaxation techniques, adequate sleep, sun exposure, and others.

A systematic review showed that psychosocial stress more than doubles the risk of hypertension, with the most related factors being post-traumatic stress disorder, anxiety and work stress [43].

On the other hand, mindfulness-based stress reduction, an example of one relaxation technique, seems to be a promising intervention and effective on the reduction of diastolic BP [44].

In conclusion, chronic anxiety and psychosocial stress can contribute to the development and control of hypertension. Managing stress is an important action to manage and control hypertension.

3. Conclusion

At the end of this review, we conclude that adopting and maintaining a healthy lifestyle pattern is a cornerstone for hypertension control. Dietary patterns including a low salt diet, weight control, exercise and physical activity, stress management, and avoiding tobacco and alcohol are all recommended to prevent, treat, and minimize morbidity and mortality secondary to hypertension.

Acknowledgements

The author would like to express his sincere gratitude to the secretary staff working at the JUST University Health Center for their support and help. The author declares that he has not received any financial support or funding for this research.

Conflict of interest

The author declares no conflict of interest.

Author details

Othman Beni Yonis
Department of Public Health and Family Medicine, Jordan University of Science and Technology (JUST University), Irbid, Jordan

*Address all correspondence to: oabaniyonis@just.edu.jo

IntechOpen

References

[1] Forouzanfar MH, Liu P, Roth GA, Ng M, Biryukov S, Marczak L, et al. Global burden of hypertension and systolic blood pressure of at least 110 to 115 mm Hg, 1990-2015. JAMA. 2017;**317**:165-182. DOI: 10.1001/jama.2016.19043

[2] Mills KT, Bundy JD, Kelly TN, Reed JE, Kearney PM, Reynolds K, et al. Global disparities of hypertension prevalence and control: A systematic analysis of population-based studies from 90 countries. Circulation. 2016;**134**:441-450. DOI: 10.1161/CIRCULATIONAHA.115.018912

[3] World Health Organization. Regional Office for the Eastern Mediterranean. Report on the regional consultation on hypertension prevention and control, Abu Dhabi, United Arab Emirates 20-22 December 2003. World Health Organization. Regional Office for the Eastern Mediterranean. 2004. Available from: https://iris.who.int/handle/10665/255066 [Accessed: April 10, 2025]

[4] Olives C, Myerson R, Mokdad AH, Murray CJL, Lim SS. Prevalence, awareness, treatment, and control of hypertension in United States counties, 2001-2009. PLoS One. 2013;**8**(4):e60308. DOI: 10.1371/journal.pone.0060308

[5] Guo F, He D, Zhang W, Walton RG. Trends in prevalence, awareness, management, and control of hypertension among United States adults, 1999 to 2010. Journal of the American College of Cardiology. 2012;**60**(7):599-606

[6] Pereira M, Lunet N, Azevedo A, Barros H. Differences in prevalence, awareness, treatment and control of hypertension between developing and developed countries. Journal of Hypertension. 2009;**27**(5):963-975

[7] Sun S et al. Gut microbiota composition and blood pressure: The CARDIA study. Hypertension. 2019;**73**(5):998-1006

[8] Grillo A et al. Sodium intake and hypertension. Nutrients. 2019;**11**(9):1970

[9] Stamler J et al. INTERSALT study findings. Public health and medical care implications. Hypertension 14.5. 1989:570-577

[10] He FJ, Li J, MacGregor GA. Effect of longer term modest salt reduction on blood pressure: Cochrane systematic review and meta-analysis of randomised trials. BMJ. 2013;**346**

[11] Halton TL, Willett WC, Liu S, Manson JE, Stampfer MJ, Hu FB. Potato and french fry consumption and risk of type 2 diabetes in women. The American Journal of Clinical Nutrition. 2006;**83**(2):284-290. DOI: 10.1093/ajcn/83.2.284

[12] Wang Q et al. Environmental ambient temperature and blood pressure in adults: A systematic review and meta-analysis. Science of the Total Environment. 2017;**575**:276-286

[13] Naja F et al. Identification of dietary patterns associated with elevated blood pressure among Lebanese men: A comparison of principal component analysis with reduced rank regression and partial least square methods. PLoS One. 2019;**14**(8):e0220942

[14] Yin X et al. Effects of salt substitutes on clinical outcomes: A systematic

review and meta-analysis. Heart. 2022;**108**(20):1608-1615

[15] Barros CL d A et al. Impact of light salt substitution for regular salt on blood pressure of hypertensive patients. Arquivos Brasileiros de Cardiologia. 2014;**104**(2):128-135

[16] Beni Yonis O et al. High rate of hypertension control among treated patients attending a teaching primary healthcare Centre in Jordan. Postgraduate Medical Journal. 2019;**95**(1122):193-197

[17] Widmer RJ, Flammer AJ, Lerman LO, Lerman A. The Mediterranean diet, its components, and cardiovascular disease. American Journal of Medicine. 2015;**128**(3):229-238. DOI: 10.1016/j. amjmed.2014.10.014. Epub 2014 Oct 15

[18] Wang H-P et al. Effect of garlic on blood pressure: A meta-analysis. The Journal of Clinical Hypertension. 2015;**17**(3):223-231

[19] Koli R, Köhler K, Tonteri E, Peltonen J, Tikkanen H, Fogelholm M. Dark chocolate and reduced snack consumption in mildly hypertensive adults: An intervention study. Nutrition Journal. 2015;**22**(14):84. DOI: 10.1186/ s12937-015-0075-3

[20] Zhang W et al. Trial of intensive blood-pressure control in older patients with hypertension. New England Journal of Medicine. 2021;**385**(14):1268-1279

[21] Barega B et al. Blood pressure control among adults with hypertension at a tertiary hospital in Ethiopia. Ethiopian Journal of Health Sciences. 2023;**33**:4

[22] Kim H-L et al. The 2022 focused update of the 2018 Korean hypertension society guidelines for the management of hypertension. Clinical Hypertension. 2023;**29**(1):11

[23] Al-Hamdan NA, Al-Zalabani AH, Saeed AA. Comparative study of physical activity of hypertensives and normotensives: A cross-sectional study of adults in Saudi Arabia. Journal of Family and Community Medicine. 2012;**19**(3):162-166

[24] Bento VFR et al. Impact of physical activity interventions on blood pressure in Brazilian populations. Arquivos Brasileiros de Cardiologia. 2015;**105**(3):301-308

[25] Dimeo F et al. Aerobic exercise reduces blood pressure in resistant hypertension. Hypertension. 2012;**60**(3):653-658

[26] Behjati Ardakani A et al. The effect of a resistance training course on blood pressure and nitric oxide levels in elderly women. Iranian Journal of Ageing. 2018;**13**(1):16-27

[27] Rasmawati R et al. Lowering blood pressure through family assistance on the implementation of self-management of hypertension elderly. Jurnal Gawat Darurat. 2022;**4**(2):129-136

[28] Juraschek SP et al. Physical fitness and hypertension in a population at risk for cardiovascular disease: The Henry ford ExercIse testing (FIT) project. Journal of the American Heart Association. 2014;**3**(6):e001268

[29] Alhomound H, Park S. Effect of bariatric surgery on hypertension. Journal of Metabolic and Bariatric Surgery. 2015;**4**(2):35-39

[30] Hedayati SS, Elsayed EF, Reilly RF. Non-pharmacological aspects of blood pressure management: What are the data? Kidney International. 2011;**79**(10):1061-1070

[31] Gilardini L et al. Effect of a modest weight loss in normalizing blood pressure

in obese subjects on antihypertensive drugs. Obesity Facts. 2016;**9**(4):251-258

[32] Soltani S et al. The effect of dietary approaches to stop hypertension (DASH) diet on weight and body composition in adults: A systematic review and meta-analysis of randomized controlled clinical trials. Obesity Reviews. 2016;**17**(5):442-454

[33] Bakre S et al. Blood pressure control in individuals with hypertension who used a digital, personalized nutrition platform: Longitudinal study. JMIR Formative Research. 2022;**6**(3):e35503

[34] Zomer E et al. Interventions that cause weight loss and the impact on cardiovascular risk factors: A systematic review and meta-analysis. Obesity Reviews. 2016;**17**(10):1001-1011

[35] Wing RR et al. Benefits of modest weight loss in improving cardiovascular risk factors in overweight and obese individuals with type 2 diabetes. Diabetes Care. 2011;**34**(7):1481-1486

[36] Kimani S et al. Association of lifestyle modification and pharmacological adherence on blood pressure control among patients with hypertension at Kenyatta National Hospital, Kenya: A cross-sectional study. BMJ Open. 2019;**9**(1):e023995

[37] Roerecke M, Kaczorowski J, Tobe SW, Gmel G, Hasan OSM, Rehm J. The effect of a reduction in alcohol consumption on blood pressure: A systematic review and meta-analysis. The Lancet Public Health. 2017;**2**(2):e108-e120. DOI: 10.1016/S2468-2667(17)30003-8. Epub 2017 Feb 7

[38] Alomari MA, Khabour OF, Alzoubi KH, Shqair DM, Eissenberg T. Central and peripheral cardiovascular changes immediately after waterpipe smoking. Inhalation Toxicology. 2014;**26**(10):579-587

[39] Cryer PE, Haymond MW, Santiago JV, Shah SD. Norepinephrine and epinephrine release and adrenergic mediation of smoking-associated hemodynamic and metabolic events. New England Journal of Medicine. 1976;**295**(11):573-577

[40] Narkiewicz K, van de Borne PJ, Hausberg M, Cooley RL, Winniford MD, Davison DE, et al. Cigarette smoking increases sympathetic outflow in humans. Circulation. 1998;**98**(6):528-534

[41] Waeber B, Schaller MD, Nussberger J, Bussien JP, Hofbauer KG, Brunner HR. Skin blood flow and cigarette smoking: The role of vasopressin. Clinical and Experimental Hypertension Part A, Theory and Practice. 1984;**6**(10-11):2003-2006

[42] Linneberg A et al. Effect of smoking on blood pressure and resting heart rate: A Mendelian randomization meta-analysis in the CARTA consortium. Circulation: Cardiovascular Genetics. 2015;**8**(6):832-841

[43] Foguet-Boreu Q, Ayerbe G-ML. Estrés psicosocial, hipertensión arterial y riesgo cardiovascular [Psychosocial stress, high blood pressure and cardiovascular risk]. Hipertens Riesgo Vascular. 2021;**38**(2):83-90. DOI: 10.1016/j.hipert.2020.09.001. Epub 2020 Oct 12

[44] Conversano C, Orrù G, Pozza A, Miccoli M, Ciacchini R, Marchi L, et al. Is mindfulness-based stress reduction effective for people with hypertension? A systematic review and meta-analysis of 30 years of evidence. International Journal of Environ Research and Public Health. 2021;**18**(6):2882. DOI: 10.3390/ijerph18062882

www.ingramcontent.com/pod-product-compliance
Lightning Source LLC
Chambersburg PA
CBHW081336190326
41458CB00018B/6020